# PRAISE FOR *A SECOND OPINION*

"In clear, eloquent prose, Relman explains how the rush to commercialize medicine harms both physicians and patients. . . . He predicts that in a decade or so, when CDHC has failed to solve the health care crisis, the country may be ready to try his plan."　　　*—Publishers Weekly*

"Highly informative, insightful and thought-provoking. It makes a very important contribution to the literature and is a must-read for anyone interested in healthcare."

*—Library Journal*

"Relman's 60 years as researcher, clinician, teacher, professional organization officer, government consultant, licensing board member, and editor in chief of the *New England Journal of Medicine* give him enormous credibility on the subject of health-care reform. . . . Everyone interested in its issues must read Relman's argument."　　　*—Booklist*

"*A Second Opinion* makes a concise, convincing case for why we need to eliminate the for-profit health care industry in the U.S. and replace it with a single-payer system."

*—Socialist Worker*

"Renowned physician, academician, and editor Arnold Relman sees the U.S. health care system as a disaster caused mainly by over-commercialization. The cure? A single-payer system. No matter where you stand on the issue, it is vital to consider Relman's potent argument and his innovative plan for change."

—STEVEN A. SCHROEDER, M.D., Distinguished Professor of Health and Healthcare, Department of Medicine, University of California, San Francisco; and former president and CEO, The Robert Wood Johnson Foundation

"*A Second Opinion* offers a lucid account of how American medicine was transformed from a professional enterprise to a business dominated by financiers. Relman, one of our most distinguished physicians and medical editors, offers reason to be optimistic about the potential for corrective action. This is a landmark contribution."

—JULIUS RICHMOND, John D. MacArthur Professor of Health Policy, Emeritus, Harvard Medical School; former Assistant Secretary of Health; and former Surgeon General of the United States

"This is a book whose importance reflects its author's credentials. Arnold Relman is an astute observer of America's health system whose understanding is enhanced by the fact that, as a physician, he has been a long time participant in its remarkable evolution. He 'cares' and, therefore, writes passionately. Yet he does so both with an historical perspective and a keen analytical eye. His years at the *New England Journal of Medicine* assure that his contribution is eminently readable. His analysis and diagnosis for what ails us should assure serious consideration both by patients and by physicians of his suggested therapy."

—RASHI FEIN, Ph.D., Professor of the Economics of Medicine, Emeritus, Harvard Medical School

# A SECOND OPINION

RESCUING AMERICA'S HEALTH CARE

A PLAN FOR UNIVERSAL COVERAGE
SERVING PATIENTS OVER PROFIT

## Arnold S. Relman, M.D.

*A Century Foundation Book*

PublicAffairs
*New York*

Hardcover first published in 2007 in the United States by
PublicAffairs™, a member of the Perseus Books Group.
Paperback first published in 2010 by PublicAffairs.
All rights reserved.
Printed in the United States of America.

PublicAffairs books are available at special discounts for bulk purchases
in the U.S. by corporations, institutions, and other organizations.
For more information, please contact the Special Markets Department
at the Perseus Books Group, 2300 Chestnut Street, Suite 200,
Philadelphia, PA 19103, or call (800) 810-4145, ext. 5000,
or e-mail special.markets@perseusbooks.com.

Book Design by Trish Wilkinson
Set in 11-point Adobe Garamond by the Perseus Books Group

The Library of Congress has cataloged the hardcover as follows:
Relman, Arnold S., 1923–
    A second opinion : how to prevent the collapse of America's
health care / Arnold S. Relman. —1st ed.
        p.   cm.
"A Century Foundation book."
    Includes bibliographical references and index.
    ISBN-13: 978-1-58648-481-1
    ISBN-10: 1-58648-481-8
    1. Health care reform—United States. I. Title.
[DNLM: 1. Health Care Reform—United States. WA 540 AA1
R3433s 2007]
RA395.A3R45 2007
362.1'0425—dc22                                    2006103332

Paperback ISBN: 978-1-58648-806-2

10 9 8 7 6 5 4 3 2 1

To M.A., of course.

# CONTENTS

# FOREWORD

THE AMERICAN WAY OF HEALTH CARE IS BOTH REVILED AND praised, sometimes by the same people. It is expensive, but it is innovative. It is unequal, but it provides some of the best care in the world. Its cost is growing far too fast for individuals and businesses, but we want even more of it. There are intense debates concerning many areas of health care—scientific issues in medical practice, prescription drugs, and emergency room use, to name a few—and underlying most of this conflict is the unusual way we pay for health care in the United States. Our approach results in our spending much more than other industrialized countries for, statistically speaking, no better results. Americans actually have been relatively passive about the considerable evidence that we are getting mediocre health care compared to other countries. Yet there is intense opposition to adaptation of the American system so that it reflects more of the efficiencies of modern European systems. At this point, the idea is politically "off the table."

Overall, however, the health care debate seems to be in a renewed stage of vitality. Given the rapid cost increases for medical procedures and coverage, the quest for a better way has become even more vigorous. As the late Herb Stein put it, "if something cannot go on forever, it will stop." Moreover, the persistence of uneven coverage makes even the most self-reliant of us uneasy, as does a steady stream of stories regarding alarmingly inefficient medical care. Adding to these concerns, the aging of the population means even greater demands for more medical services. The debate over health care is likely to be at or near the top of the public agenda for the foreseeable future.

In most of the developed world, universal health care coverage is standard. The question is, how long will the United States remain the outlier from this pattern? While the debate about universal health care has been revived in this country, it remains too early to judge whether it will gain the momentum needed to overturn considerable political resistance and enormous practical questions. The fact that 46 million Americans are uninsured ought to provoke a powerful call for action. Perhaps this is just a measure of the limited political clout held by this portion of the population, but it should be cause for great concern, because it affects costs for everyone. Because the uninsured often seek uncompensated care through emergency rooms, the financial burden of these services is transferred to current payers into the system in the form of higher costs.

While there is movement underway in Massachusetts, California, and other states to provide universal health care, since the failure of the Clinton health care plan of the 1990s, proposals for sweeping health care reform at the federal level have been scarce. But this long-dormant debate seems likely to break out again, as some members of Congress have pledged to take on the problem. There will be fierce resistance from some quarters, but the time has come for a fresh discussion of the American form of health care.

In that sense, a book by Dr. Arnold Relman, the distinguished former editor of the *New England Journal of Medicine*, could not be more timely. Over two decades ago, Relman coined the phrase "medical industrial complex" to describe the "recent relatively unheralded rise of the new industry that supplies health care services for profit." He feared that this industry would worsen the problems of overuse and fragmentation of medical services, lead to overemphasis on using new medical technology, and unduly influence debates over national health policy. In this book, Relman finds that his predictions have been borne out and that the influence of what one writer calls "money-driven medicine" has increased dramatically. He offers evidence to refute the claims of for-profit medicine to greater efficiency; he doubts that health savings accounts and other "consumer-driven" plans will lower costs and reduce the number of uninsured. Relman proposes a bold single-payer model for universal coverage, combined with a not-for-profit system for the delivery of medical care that is based on prepaid multi-specialty group practices and salaried physicians. He believes that reform of the insurance system will not control rising costs without a major change in the organization of medical practice and the payment of physicians. He also calls on doctors to reclaim their roles as counselors to patients and managers of clinical decision-making and to jumpstart the reform campaign.

This single-payer model, of course, is just one of several approaches that need to be considered as the health care conversation deepens and sharpens in the United States. At The Century Foundation, we have published numerous works related to this field in recent years, including David J. Rothman's *Beginnings Count: The Technological Imperative in American Healthcare; Too Much of a Good thing? Why Healthcare Spending Won't Make Us Sick,* and *Apart at the Seams: The Collapse of Private Pension and Healthcare Protections,* both by Charles R. Morris; *Medicare Tomorrow: The Report of the Century Foundation Task Force on Medicare Reform;* and *A New Deal for Health: How to Cover Everyone and Get Medical Costs under Control,* by Leif Wellington Haase.

We continue working under the leadership of our health care fellow, Leif Wellington Haase, on approaches that would provide coverage for all Americans and expect to produce additional reports in the months and years to come. In this context, Dr. Relman's thoughtful contribution is especially welcome. He has been a major figure in the medical field—his personal views are invaluable because they have been formulated during a lifetime of science and experience. In his discussion of the market's inability to provide virtuous results in health care, he addresses the big questions in a bold and accessible way.

On behalf of the trustees of The Century Foundation, I thank him for this important contribution to one of the nation's most important public policy debates.

Richard C. Leone, *President*
The Century Foundation

# PREFACE

## Why a "Second Opinion?"

Our health care system is failing us badly, as almost everyone knows. The evidence has been described and analyzed endlessly in the popular media and in the health policy literature. In the past decade alone, scores of books on the subject have been published, so it would seem there couldn't be much more to say.

Why, then, would I venture to add yet another book to this multitude? I suppose the most honest answer is that I felt compelled to. My experience has been quite different from that of most other authors writing about the health care system. It has led me to a different view of what is wrong and what needs to be done. Given the importance of health care for the public, I wanted that viewpoint to reach as wide an audience as possible.

Books about the health care system are usually written by economists, social scientists, or business experts, and naturally, their perspective is shaped by their own disciplines. Physicians, with a few notable exceptions, are too occupied with the demands of clinical practice to have the time to write books about the system in which they work. So the task has largely been left to others outside of medicine, despite the fact that the health care system is mainly about doctors and patients and the care of the sick.

In my long life as a physician, I have been privileged to serve in many capacities. I have been a research scientist, a clinician, a medical school teacher and department head, a university trustee, an officer of professional organizations, a consultant to government, the editor of an influential medical journal, and a member of a state board of licensure and discipline. Although I claim no special wisdom as a result, the breadth and depth of this experience has provided an unusual opportunity to study U.S. medicine up close in all its aspects, and to participate in some of the important developments that have changed the practice and financing of medical care over the past half century. This experience has brought me to my present ideas about the health care system, its problems, and their solution. Most of these ideas differ from currently popular views.

Shortly after becoming editor of the *New England Journal of Medicine* in 1977, I began to realize that as vast new funds were moving into medical care, the health care system was rapidly changing from a professional service primarily devoted to the care of the sick into a lucrative and competitive marketplace for investors and investor-owned corporations. Not-for-profit facilities and practicing physicians were also being drawn into the competition for income and market share. Investor-owned health insurance companies were entering this market, as well, and an enormous new industry was taking shape. I worried that this commercialization of medicine would have serious consequences for the cost, quality, and accessibility of medical care, and for the ethical foundations of the medical profession and the institutional providers of care.

I first wrote about this in the *New England Journal of Medicine* in 1980, referring to the emerging system as "the medical-industrial complex," and have published many articles on the subject since. A large body of literature has generally confirmed the facts that I first noted more than a quarter century ago, but most authors have not shared my interpretation of these facts or my ideas about the widespread policy changes they call for. A common view is that piecemeal reform, a change in market strategy, or some readjustments in tax policies are all the present system needs. Economists in particular argue that most of the health care system's problems can be solved simply by allowing the market to work, with only minimal help from government.

My experience has convinced me otherwise. I can't accept any of these views because they start with a misunderstanding of the essential nature of medical care, of the prime purpose of a health care system, and of the basic causes of our current problems. What follows is a "second opinion" about the state of our health care system and the major reforms it requires. It is in essence a personal manifesto. Because it deals with important practical issues about health care in the United States that should be of concern to everyone, it is written for the general reader. However, I also include an "open letter" to physicians, because they have a central role in health care and must be involved in the planning and implementation of any reform.

The literature on the topics covered in this book is enormous; no attempt has been made to review it. That would be quite impossible and would serve no useful purpose here. What I have done, instead, is to cite only a few of the most significant articles and then mention general references that readers seeking more information on a particular subject can consult. Those citations, plus some additional documentation and a certain amount of commentary that supplements the text, are all to be found in the notes. Hoping that you will read both the text and the notes in their entirety, I have made both as brief as possible.

If I have done my task properly, you will be interested enough in the book's message to want a wide public debate on the issues it raises. And if I have done my job really well, you may even be persuaded that the reforms I propose are necessary, feasible, and worth supporting.

# INTRODUCTION

> The U.S. health care system becomes a more embarrassing disaster each year . . .
>
> —DONALD KENNEDY, FORMER PRESIDENT,
> STANFORD UNIVERSITY; EDITOR-IN-CHIEF,
> *SCIENCE*, AUGUST 15, 2003

> America has the best health care system in the world, pure and simple.
>
> —PRESIDENT GEORGE W. BUSH, ADDRESSING THE
> AMERICAN HOSPITAL ASSOCIATION, MAY 1, 2006

AMERICA'S HEALTH CARE SYSTEM IS MUCH TOO EXPENSIVE, AND its costs are rising at an unsustainable rate. Furthermore, care is not available to many who need it the most, and it is inefficient and highly variable in quality.

Failure to provide health insurance coverage for all is sometimes seen as our most important problem, but high costs are really at the heart of the U.S. dilemma. The financial burden of insurance is straining our resources, and the cost of achieving universal coverage appears to make that objective impossible.[1] We spend much more on health care than any other country in the world, whether expressed per capita or as a fraction of our total economy, but by most measures of national health, we rank well below many other advanced countries that spend less and still manage to cover almost all of their citizens.[2] Total U.S. expenditures are now over $2 trillion per year, or over 16 percent of our gross national product. Yet over 15 percent of our people are uninsured, and this percentage increases each year.[3] Many of the rest are underinsured, with often disastrous consequences for their health and financial stability. Health care costs are a common cause of family financial difficulties and personal bankruptcy, and they are a major economic threat to the viability of many businesses. High costs are forcing a growing number of Americans to seek treatment in Asian countries such as India, Singapore, and Thailand, where medical services are much cheaper than in the United States.

What makes U.S. health care so much more expensive than even that of other western countries? I believe it is the extent to which the insurance and delivery of our medical care is governed by commerce and private enterprise rather than by public regulation and social need.

Whereas most western countries have public or government-regulated health insurance programs that cover most or all of their population, only about one-third of U.S. citizens have that kind of coverage. Whatever insurance the rest may have is provided through hundreds of private plans, most of which are for-profit businesses. In most other western countries, the majority of health care facilities are publicly owned, but in the United States most facilities are private, and often for-profit. Within the United States, the overall practice of medicine is more entrepreneurial than elsewhere. Our physicians are more specialized, more likely to be paid on a fee-for-service basis, and more likely to have financial interests in health care facilities and products than physicians in most other western countries. Business incentives dominate our system, influencing the behavior of all facilities, for-profit and not-for-profit alike, as well as the behavior of physicians. Our health care system tends to emphasize income and profits over social utility or the efficient use of resources. When insurers and providers focus on maximizing their income, health care expenditures inevitably rise, equity is neglected, and quality of care suffers.

Considering its high cost, mediocre performance, and failure to provide universal care, it should be no surprise that most people agree our present health care system is seriously flawed and must change.[4] But that is where agreement ends. The many different proposed alternative plans have focused variously on the funding and insurance systems, or the delivery system, or the so-called marketplace in which these systems operate, but almost never on the holistic structure of health care.

I believe that only a comprehensive approach, aimed at improving all aspects of the system, is likely to be successful in achieving a long-term solution. *To develop a health care system that covers everyone and provides good quality care at a cost we can afford to live with, we need to change not only our system of insuring and paying for health care but also the way we organize and deliver that care.* I am convinced that within a decade or so, we will begin to see drastic reforms of this kind because the present commercialized system cannot last much longer and incremental improvements will be of little avail. Our health care system is in a tailspin, and only major reform will prevent its impending crash. Now is the time to reassess our situation. We should be asking what we have learned from our problems with the health care system over the past few decades, and how the lessons of this unhappy experience can be applied to our efforts at reform.

Major reform will require public understanding of our basic problems. There is much popular misinformation and confusion about our health care system and the options for reform. Some of this confusion is deliberately generated by the entrenched commercial interests that want no change, and some of it is advanced by those who see only a market-based solution. It is difficult for the uninformed outsider to understand how the health care system works and to separate myths and self-serving claims from reality. A major objective of this book, therefore, is to dispel confusion and help readers understand the key facts and issues that demand new policies. When reduced to its essentials, the health care system is not that difficult to comprehend, making possible remedies easier to evaluate.

This book attempts to explain why piecemeal marginal improvements won't support our present system much longer, and why continued or even greater reliance on the market will be disastrous. It offers an analysis of what has gone wrong with U.S. health care over the past few decades and what needs to be done to correct it. It does not pretend to solve *all* the problems that block the road to reform, but it does offer explanations and suggests remedies for much of what currently ails our system. At the least, I hope it will provide readers with the background information to make their own decisions about health care reform and the need for political action.

The book has six chapters that deal with the present system and its reform, each intended to build on the one before. Because our system is so often compared with Canada's, which is frequently offered as a model, a seventh chapter concerns the present problems of the Canadian system and what they can teach us. The final chapter is directed toward physicians, who too often have been part of the problem, not the solution. I am convinced that no worthwhile reform of U.S. health care will occur without the active participation of its doctors.

## Summary of Chapters

To guide the reader through the argument of the book, which is contained in Chapters 1–6, I offer summaries of these chapters below, followed by brief descriptions of Chapters 7 and 8, the two supplementary chapters. Readers who may want to sample chapters out of order or go directly to my discussion of a topic of particular interest to them can do so after reading these summaries. For most readers, however, I recommend reading the first six chapters in the usual manner from beginning to end, because it may be difficult to follow the exposition in places without having read what has preceded it.

Chapter 1, "The Commercialization of U.S. Medicine," begins with a brief history of the remarkable, recent commercialization of our health care system. Too many people are simply unaware of this history. And yet without knowing it, one cannot understand why and how the system was transformed so dramatically during the first few decades after World War II. I tell this story from the perspective of a physician who lived through these changes and was personally involved in many of them.

I consider the transformation of the U.S. health care system from a professional service for the sick and injured into one of the country's largest industries to be the most important socioeconomic change in the last half century of health care in our country. This transformation occurred against the background of a great postwar expansion of third-party indemnification insurance. ("Third-party" refers to payers other than patients themselves and "indemnification" means insurance that pays the itemized charges of the providers.) There was also a rapid increase in the number of physicians, hospitals, and clinical facilities of all kinds. This was a time when many new medical centers—meaning a medical school with other health professions schools and one or more adjacent teaching hospitals—were built. This period also saw an extraordinary growth in basic and applied medical research, leading to new technology, new treatments, and the rise of new medical and surgical specialties. Today, the number of specialists has grown and now exceeds the number of primary care physicians. All of these developments were important in creating the conditions that made the commercial transformation possible and financially attractive to insurers and providers, but commercialization was the catalyst that changed the whole U.S. health system into a de facto industry. Commercialization, with its incentives to maximize revenues, provided the energy to ignite an explosion of expenditures on health care that is now consuming so much of our economy.

Private commerce, largely free from government regulation, made health care in our country different from that in the rest of the Western world. The expansion and technological development of health services in the United States was inevitable and occurred in all advanced countries. The same can be said about the growth of health insurance, but not about commercialization. Commercial development was for a long time largely confined to the United States, although it has recently begun to marginally affect the health systems of other advanced countries as well.

Commercialization of health care in the United States created what I termed "the New Medical-Industrial Complex" in a 1980 article in the *New England Journal of Medicine*. I was referring to a medical care system that had begun to attract investors, and in which business interests had started to reshape the behavior of doctors and health care facilities. At the time I wrote this, the phrase "health care industry" sounded odd to most people, but now it is taken for granted. However, the basic purpose of medical care is fundamentally different from that of a business transaction, despite the fact that most physicians earn their living, and most facilities are supported through income generated by the provision of that care. Nevertheless, market forces, investors, for-profit corporations, and entrepreneurs are now at the center of the U.S. system, and generation of income is a dominant consideration for most private providers of health care—including those that are not investor owned. So the history I tell in this chapter is largely focused on these questions: How and why did the U.S. "medical-industrial complex" arise, and what drew investors to the health care system?

Chapter 2, "The Consequences of Commercialized Care," deals with the consequences of the commercial and technological transformation of health care in the United States. Other factors played a role, but I contend that this transformation, coupled with a largely open-ended fee-for-service insurance payment system, is primarily responsible for today's problems. I explain why our commercialized health care system is beset with uncontrollable costs, why it fails to provide adequate insurance coverage for so many, why medical services are so erratically and inequitably distributed, and why their quality is so variable and so often substandard. I argue that these problems and the general public discontent with the system are largely the predictable results of allowing market principles to shape our national health care policies and of permitting economic forces to determine the behavior of health care institutions and medical practitioners.

This chapter also summarizes the few apparently reliable empirical studies comparing for-profit and not-for-profit care in the United States. Almost all of this evidence supports the conclusion that business ownership of health care facilities is more expensive and less efficient than non-profit ownership (that is, has higher overhead and administrative costs), despite all the mythology to the contrary, and that it delivers services of no better—and sometimes inferior—quality. Of course, this empirical evidence does not demonstrate that not-for-profit care itself is as good or efficient as it should be. "Not-for-profit" does not mean "not-for-income." The commercial transformation of health care has affected the behavior of almost all private institutions providing health care, regardless of whether they pay taxes. So the fact that not-for-profit facilities seem to outperform their investor-owned rivals in the comparisons described here should not conceal the fact that income maximization is a powerful incentive throughout the entire health system and often creates a conflict between the financial interests of the provider and the health needs of the patient. The chapter ends with a brief consideration of the role of physicians in generating health care costs.

Chapter 3, "The Revolt of the Payers," describes how government and private insurers (the "payers") have tried to contain rising costs for the past few decades and why these efforts have been unsuccessful, or at best unsustainable. My contention is that attempts to control medical cost inflation have in the end failed because they have not dealt with its underlying causes, which are as much on the delivery side of the care system as on the insurance and funding side. "Managed care," HMOs (health maintenance organizations), and fee schedules for hospitals and physicians based on diagnosis-related groups (DRGs) and a relative value scale (RBRVS) respectively, have not been successful in containing costs, because they have had relatively little sustained effect on the motivation and behavior of physicians and health care facilities. They have concentrated on the payment and insurance of care and not on the delivery of services. Furthermore, these approaches have antagonized patients, doctors, and most health care facilities. In 1993, the new Clinton administration proposed an elaborate new system based on "managed competition" among private HMOs, with a cap on total expenditures to control costs. Whatever its virtues, the proposal was too complicated to be easily understood by nonexperts and involved more government regulation than most businesspeople could abide. Within a year after its proposal, it died in congressional committee without ever coming to a floor vote, defeated by vested business interests, political partisans opposing "big government," and the opposition of the medical profession.

For a few years during the mid-1990s, HMOs managed to stabilize expenditures in the private sector, but backlash from patients and physicians forced employers to change from HMOs to less controlling forms of insurance. By the turn of the century, private costs had resumed their escalation in parallel with the steadily rising costs of Medicare and Medicaid. In response, both public and private insurers have been shifting an increasing fraction of the burden of payment to their beneficiaries, while employment-related programs have been steadily reducing their benefits and the number of beneficiaries covered. The failure of HMOs and their version of managed care to control insurance premiums for more than a few years has led to proposals for other approaches. Rationing, elimination of costly diseases through application of new medical science, reform of the malpractice system, and the moderation of expectations for unlimited medical care have all been suggested as cost-control measures. But they cannot do the job, as I explain.

Chapter 4, "'Consumer-Driven' Health Care: The New New Thing," covers the latest and most widely touted effort at moderating the rise of medical costs through "market-based" or "consumer-driven" health care (CDHC). It is being promoted as part of a new trend called the "ownership society," which purports to give "consumers" (that is, patients) a larger stake in managing their own care and give providers greater scope for competition. CDHC, which gives more responsibility to patients for selecting their care and bearing its costs, is now the fashionable trend in health policy.

Based on high-deductible insurance for catastrophic costs that is coupled with individually owned "health savings accounts," CDHC plans currently constitute only a small fraction of private insurance, covering only a few million people. However, they are spreading rapidly and could become a major part of the private insurance system, and a significant fraction of public insurance plans as well. This chapter examines the implications of this approach to health insurance and shows why it is basically unfair and unrealistic, and is unlikely to work. It probably won't control costs, but it could undermine the social values of health insurance and aggravate the fragmentation and incoordination of care. Nevertheless, the influence of market-based ideology is now so widespread that CDHC, and other similar methods of shifting more responsibility to patients for choosing and financing their own care, will probably continue to expand before they are finally rejected. Just as HMOs did, CDHC will have to play itself out before attention can be given to other policy alternatives. The myth that "competitive markets" and more active "consumers" can cure our health system's problems will die hard, but it is fundamentally inconsistent with the realities of medical care and therefore is doomed to fail.

Chapter 5, "The Reform We Need," suggests that after "market-based" policies fail, pressure for major reform will rapidly increase. In this chapter I propose a reformed system that I believe would work. It includes changes in the insurance and delivery systems that could control the inflation of costs, while providing universal coverage and improving the quality of care. The plan would include a simplified, single-payer insurance system, which would provide everyone with a standard package of benefits, including acute and chronic care. Amenities and services not covered by the system could be purchased out-of-pocket or paid through additional private insurance. The universal insurance system would be funded through a graduated earmarked health care tax and administered by a public-private health agency, like the Federal Reserve Board. Cost would not be an impediment in adopting this plan because we already spend enough to pay for all medically justifiable care, without much, if any, additional funds. The public and private money now being spent on health insurance would need to be pooled, redirected to an efficient central insurer, and distributed to a reorganized and largely not-for-profit system for medical care.

The delivery of most ambulatory medical care would be through not-for-profit multi-specialty medical groups, paid in advance on a per capita basis. These groups would be privately managed, and physicians would largely be paid through salaries determined by the management of the groups, but legally limited in total to a specified percentage of the gross income of the group. Hospitals and other facilities providing services under the national insurance plan could be paid through budgets negotiated with the health agency, but I favor paying facilities with standardized fees from the practice groups. In any case, all such facilities would be not-for-profit and, like the group practices, would be held harmless by the central fund for losses due to caring for very sick patients. More rational use of technology by physicians would be facilitated by the elimination of fee-for-service payment and by a national system for technology evaluation and outcome reporting.

This new approach to funding, insuring, and delivering health care is described only in broad strokes, as I recognize that many details would have to be worked out or modified by later experience. My purpose here is simply to demonstrate the logic and financial feasibility of the reform plan and suggest that its objectives could probably be achieved without spending much additional money—given the political will to implement it.

Chapter 6, "Can We Get There? Do We Want To?" considers the practical problems of achieving the kind of reform proposed in Chapter 5. It acknowledges that the hurdles are formidable and that a gradual, stepwise approach may be required. However, ultimate success is likely if the reform plan is actively supported by the public and the medical profession. Opposition from the vested economic interests of the "medical-industrial complex" could be neutralized by the opposed economic interests of employers, as they come to realize that they have more to gain from this kind of major reform than from any other approach to controlling their health care expenses. And ideological resistance among legislators to a publicly funded and regulated health care system would ultimately fade when they realize that there is no other practical way to avoid the budget-busting consequences of uncontrollable health costs. In any case, constituent votes carry more weight with legislators than the efforts of lobbyists or the financial contributions of the industries that will oppose reform. If it becomes clear that voters demand reform and if, as Chapter 5 demonstrates, reform does not require much new federal money, then legislative action could follow.

Chapter 7, "Lessons from Canada," gives a brief overview of Canada's approach to health care insurance, explaining the important differences and similarities between our two systems. I discuss Canada's current problems because the Canadian public Medicare system is so often compared with our own mix of public and private programs. Unlike other countries with government-supported health insurance, Canada's health care system was very similar to ours for many years, so its relatively recent experience with a universal system is often cited in discussions of single-payer reform in the United States. Current proposals to increase the privatization of the Canadian system have attracted much attention from U.S. health care pundits. I explain the reasons for recent criticisms of the Canadian system and for the move toward private facilities outside the public system, and I suggest how our experience might hold some solutions for Canada. I also propose that incorporation of some key features of the Canadian system into our own might be just what we need.

In the final analysis, however, the most important lesson is that differences in the health care systems in two advanced countries such as the United States and Canada inevitably reflect differences in political values and national will. In neither country has the medical profession contributed all it could to the solution of the health care system's most pressing problems. Certainly in the United States, physicians have too often been part of the system's problems instead of working constructively on solutions.

In Chapter 8, "An Open Letter to My Colleagues in the Medical Profession," I urge physicians to take up the cause of major reform.

I remind them that their traditional resistance to change has not served them or their patients very well. Practicing physicians were essentially uninvolved in the planning for the health initiative proposed by the Clinton administration in 1993, and this was an important (but not the only) reason for its defeat. No future reform is likely to be enacted, or at least implemented, without substantial support from the profession. Inasmuch as the reform needed now must involve major changes in the delivery as well as the insurance of health care, I argue that the profession must not only abandon its historical resistance to such reform but needs to play a major part in planning for a new system and making it work.

The present control of medical practice by market economics does not serve the health care needs of patients very well and is not compatible with a strong, ethically based profession. Practice under such circumstances cannot meet the expectations that have traditionally drawn young people to medical careers. If the market continues to prevail, medicine will lose much of its appeal as an honorable profession committed to serving the needs of the sick— and this is what has attracted the best students. However, contrary to the conventional views of most experts, I believe that strong forces for reform will within a decade or so create an opportunity to reverse this trend. Much of what happens then will depend on how effectively the medical profession becomes involved in planning for change.

I urge physicians not only to support the development of a single-payer insurance system, but to help devise the reforms in the delivery system that must accompany single-payer insurance, if inflation in medical costs is to be controlled and quality of care improved. The key to this new delivery system should be the development of prepaid multi-specialty medical groups in which physicians are paid largely by salary. I explain how such groups would improve patient care, encourage professional values, and make physicians' lives more satisfying. I end by suggesting that the hour is late if physicians want to continue to be advocates and counselors for patients. Unless we physicians help to devise a better health care system, we are likely to become little more than highly trained, specialized workers in a system dominated by corporations or government.

# 1

# THE COMMERCIALIZATION
# OF U.S. MEDICINE

The business of America is business.
—President Calvin Coolidge

The U.S. health care system is now commonly called an "industry," and in many ways that is an apt description. A large proportion of its privately owned institutions and facilities are for-profit businesses, or behave as if they were. For them, maximizing income can take priority over serving the medical needs of sick people, especially when those sick people are poor. Even though physicians have traditionally held themselves to be professionals rather than tradespeople, many now regard their practices as a form of business and engage in activities best described as entrepreneurial.

Publicly traded, investor-owned businesses abound in our health care system today. They are not simply firms that market products and supporting services like drugs, medical equipment, or hospital supplies, but businesses that design and provide health insurance and manage or deliver the care. The latter functions were formerly performed almost entirely on a not-for-profit basis. Now they are often sold for profit by investor-owned corporations whose fiduciary responsibility is to maximize profits for stockholders. No other health care system in the world is commercialized to that extent.

To understand how we got here, we need to look back about sixty years. To some degree, the forces that created our present system were already at work before then, but the story I want to tell begins just after World War II. The war stimulated a major expansion of U.S. medicine, which then set the stage for its later commercial transformation. The end of the war also happens to be the time when I entered medicine.

I graduated from medical school in 1946, when the medical profession looked very different. There were only about 140 doctors per 100,000 people; since then, that number has nearly doubled. In 1946, most physicians were in solo office practice or shared an office with a few partners. Most doctors were in primary care—as general practitioners or general internists. Specialists constituted only about one-third of all doctors, among whom general surgeons, pediatricians, ophthalmologists, and obstetrician-gynecologists were the most numerous. The other now numerous specialties were either a much smaller fraction of the physician population or didn't yet exist. Today, almost two-thirds of physicians are specialists or subspecialists. In 1946, only a few percent of practitioners were women. Now, almost 30 percent are women, and that percentage is rising rapidly because about half of all students entering U.S. medical schools are women. There were only a handful of large multi-specialty group practices in 1946, most of which were in the Midwest and Far West. Now, there are over 300 multi-specialty group practices that are members of the American Medical Group Association (the trade association for group practices in the United States). These groups have an estimated 82,000 physicians on their staff, and they are located throughout the country.[1]

The hospital system was also different. In the late nineteenth and early twentieth centuries, there were many small hospitals owned by the physicians who practiced in them. By the 1930s and 1940s, they were replaced by larger facilities owned by boards of trustees, church groups, or government at all levels. When I graduated from medical school, almost all the acute care general hospitals were independent not-for-profit institutions, and the total number of hospital beds was about 350 per 100,000 people. The number of hospital beds had increased to over 400 per 100,000 by 1980, but since then has fallen to little more than 300 per 100,000. The most significant change in hospitals since I entered the profession has been the appearance, beginning in the 1960s, of chains of investor-owned hospitals, a phenomenon discussed later in this chapter.

The kind of medical care provided in 1946 was also vastly different. It was much simpler, less expensive—and less effective. It consisted mostly of individual transactions between physicians and patients, which took place in patients' homes, doctors' offices, or not-for-profit hospitals and clinics. Patients were rarely referred to specialists, and only a few of these referrals resulted in the use of expensive technology or specialized facilities. Physicians used a very small number of patented pharmaceuticals, and they were relatively inexpensive. Much pharmacotherapy involved generic drugs or non-patented ingredients that were prepared and dispensed by pharmacists according to physicians' prescriptions. Total expenditures for medical care were less than 4 percent of the economy, and government paid for less than 20 percent of that, mainly for veterans, government employees, military and public health services, and city and county hospitals and clinics.

Although some privately purchased insurance for hospital bills and for doctors' services had been available through Blue Cross and Blue Shield associations even before World War II, the great majority of Americans in 1946 were uninsured. They paid their medical bills out of pocket if they could afford to. If not, they had to rely on the charity of physicians and community institutions or on government-supported hospitals and clinics. This by no means ensured that the poor were adequately treated. But they could usually get emergency care or minimal continuing care in private community or public tax-supported hospitals, or in the offices of physicians who considered this to be part of their professional obligation. Then, as now, being poor meant that you were much less likely to receive all the care you needed.

The prevailing view in 1946 was that the practice of medicine was a profession, not a business. It was generally held that physicians, as professionals, had a responsibility to attend to the medical needs of all who consulted them, and to put that obligation before considerations of financial gain. That isn't to say physicians weren't at all concerned about their livelihood. They were, and they could expect to earn a good living as a reward for their hard work. They could pretty well count on doing so, because there were only half as many practicing physicians per population as there are now, and most doctors in urban and suburban areas had all the paying patients they could handle. However, financial success was not the paramount ambition for the great majority of my contemporaries.

Most of the administrators who managed hospitals in the late 1940s didn't think that maximizing the institution's income was a primary goal, either. Hospitals were not thought to be businesses in the usual sense. Since most of them were owned by voluntary boards of trustees or church-related groups or government, they were expected to meet the medical needs of their communities.

Few people thought of health care as a market for investment. Investors were not interested in health care services, although they did invest in drug companies and other businesses that manufactured medical supplies and equipment. The delivery of medical care by physicians and hospitals in the 1940s was not only a relatively insignificant part of the national economy, it was not even considered to be a commercial enterprise.

If anyone had used the term "health care industry" in 1946, few would have known what that meant. The language, attitudes, and values of health care providers reflected those of a social service, not a business. In short, our health care system had not yet become "monetarized."[2] Although U.S. society did not at the time ensure universal access to health care (and still does not), most physicians I knew believed they were providing a necessary service that ought to be available to everyone who needed it, regardless of ability to pay. As the sociologist Paul Starr (no apologist for the medical profession) wrote in his 1982 classic study, *The Social Transformation of American Medicine*, "The organizational culture of medicine used to be dominated by the ideals of professionalism and voluntarism, which softened the underlying acquisitive activity."[3]

The great majority of my classmates expected to end up in private office practice. A few, like me, hoped to become academics, who could enjoy combined careers in practice, teaching, and research as a member of a medical school faculty. These aspirations were encouraged by the dramatic scientific changes in U.S. medicine that were beginning at about that time. The construction after World War II of a huge new research campus for the National Institutes of Health (NIH) in Bethesda, Maryland, and the rapid expansion of government support for medical research and education led to the development of many new drugs and technologies, new treatments and diagnostic tests, and the growth of new medical specialties. Federal and state money subsidized the construction of new medical schools and hospitals, and the expansion and renovation of older institutions. As a result, more students were entering medical school, and more were becoming specialists and sub-specialists.

## The Postwar Transformation of Medicine

The story of the burgeoning growth of U.S. medical research and education in the years following World War II and the resulting transformation in the practice of medicine is familiar enough.[4] It occurred to a varying degree in all advanced countries, but the United States led the world. There is no need to retell this story in

any detail here, except to note that the resulting expansion of technology, specialized medical personnel, new facilities, and expensive
medical services of all kinds were essential to the subsequent commercialization of medicine in the United States.

The other key element was the rapid postwar expansion of medical insurance, in part a response to the growing expense of the more
sophisticated medical services. In turn, insurance stimulated the provision of still more services and the expenditure of more money on
medical care. Although there was some private insurance that covered the costs of physicians' services and hospital care even before the
war, it mainly consisted of not-for-profit Blue Cross (hospital insurance) and Blue Shield plans (insurance for physicians' services) and a
few plans offered by commercial insurance companies. But it was
not until after the war that private medical insurance really took off.

Most of the postwar expansion of private insurance came from
coverage provided to workers and their families by large employers.[5]
This fringe benefit, which was tax free to workers and tax deductible
for employers, was regarded as equivalent to wage increases (which
had been frozen by law during the war). It was negotiated annually
with employers by the unions and soon came to be a critical element
in collective bargaining. Employers selected insurance plans and the
benefits available to their employees—often only the one or two
plans considered by management to offer the best deal at the best
prices. Most plans required a contribution to the premium (about
20 percent) from employees. Employers usually purchased coverage
from private insurance companies for premiums that were negotiated, but some employers (usually the largest) acted as their own insurers so that their expenses varied with the health needs of their
workers. These large employers used insurance companies only for
administration, for paying health care bills, and for review of claims.

At first, most of the insurers paid doctors and hospitals on an "indemnity" basis; that is, the providers of care submitted itemized bills
and were reimbursed on a "cost-plus" basis. "Cost plus" meant that

providers usually set their own charges, based on their costs plus a "usual and customary" profit. In essence, the insurers paid whatever the doctors and hospitals asked. In the early phase of employment-based insurance, the only exceptions to this rule were the few large prepaid health plans like Kaiser-Permanente, Group Health of Puget Sound, and the Health Insurance Plan (HIP) in New York. These organizations were in effect the earliest postwar HMOs because they combined insurance with the delivery of medical care. For a prepaid annual premium, they offered employers a defined package of medical services for their employees, provided by a large multi-specialty group of physicians. If they could provide care for less than the premiums, they could keep the surplus; if it cost them more, they had to recoup the loss when renegotiating the premium for the following year. Premiums for all types of private insurance steadily rose to cover the constantly rising per capita costs of health care.

By 1957, 12 million employees and 20 million dependents had employment-based insurance, and these numbers continued to increase rapidly until recently. Today, nearly 160 million people, including retired workers and their dependents, are covered, but the number of insured individuals is dwindling, as employers, hard pressed by rising costs, seek relief from this burden by eliminating coverage for dependents and relying more on temporary workers who do not qualify for insurance benefits. Employers are also shifting more responsibility for payment to their employees, thus forcing an increasing number to decline coverage. Between the years 2000 and 2005, approximately 5 million employees lost their insurance, and most of those who are still insured pay more toward the cost of their premiums.[6]

## Enter the Economists

The early growth of private health insurance during the decades of the 1940s and 1950s attracted the attention of only a few economists, whose discipline had until then largely ignored health care. Of particular interest to the early health care economists were workforce issues and theoretical questions about the pricing of premiums and the so-called moral hazard (the insured beneficiary's temptation to overuse services not paid out of pocket) created by indemnity-type insurance and first-dollar coverage.

The field of health economics was still struggling to define itself when, in 1963, a seminal article was published in the *American Economic Review* by Kenneth J. Arrow of Stanford University.[7] Arrow was later to share the Nobel Prize in 1972 for his theoretical work in microeconomics. This article, although concerned mainly with the economic theory of health insurance, offered important observations on medical care as a market. Arrow argued that the medical care system was set apart from other markets by several unique characteristics, including: (1) a demand for services that was irregular and unpredictable, and often associated with what he called an "assault on personal integrity," because it frequently arose from life-threatening illness or injury; (2) a supply of services that did not simply respond to the desires of buyers but was mainly determined by the professional judgment of physicians about the medical needs of their patients (Arrow pointed out that doctors differ from vendors of most other services because they are expected by the norms of their profession to place a primary concern for their patients' medical needs above considerations of profit); (3) limitations on the entry of providers into the market, resulting from the high costs and exacting standards of medical education and professional licensure; and (4) insensitivity to prices and a near absence of price competition.

Perhaps the most incisive of Arrow's insights was his recognition of what he called the "uncertainty" inherent in medical care. By this he meant the great asymmetry of information between provider and buyer concerning the need for, and the probable consequences of, a particular medical service or course of action. Patients usually know much less about the diagnosis and treatment of their disease or injury than their doctors do. Furthermore, because of illness or injury they may be in no condition to evaluate their options. As a consequence they cannot independently decide what medical services they want in the same way consumers choose services in the usual market, shopping for what they want, at the prices they are willing to pay. The penalties for making a mistake in the health care market are usually higher than in others. Patients must therefore trust their physicians to decide, or at least recommend, what services they need. Arrow concluded that to protect the interests of patients in such circumstances, society must rely on nonmarket mechanisms (such as professional educational standards, and state licensure) rather than on the discipline of the market and the choices of informed buyers.

Arrow's analysis could logically have led to the further conclusion that the medical care system is not really a market at all, and that therefore much economic theory is largely irrelevant to discussions of health care policy. However, for reasons I will explain below, the market view of health care soon prevailed. Now, in our current business-oriented society, it is widely assumed that market theory applies to virtually all human activity involving the exchange of goods and services for money, and this dogma is rarely questioned.

In the years since Arrow's article appeared, health economics has grown into a large and influential subdiscipline of economics, and economic analysis has played an important role in shaping health care policy in both the public and private sector.[8] I believe it is fair to say that today most economists think medical care is indeed a market, although admittedly imperfect and idiosyncratic, and that it should thus obey economic theory.[9]

## The Coming of Medicare and Medicaid

Arrow's paper is generally acknowledged to have been a landmark in the early literature of health economics. It might have had more influence on the subsequent discussions of U.S. health policy, if not for the birth of Medicare and Medicaid, which dramatically changed the landscape of health care. In 1965, the newly elected administration of Lyndon B. Johnson was determined to use the majority it held in both houses of Congress, along with the nation's grief over the assassination of John F. Kennedy, to push through some of the social reforms Kennedy had not been able to achieve during his brief tenure. Although employment-based private health insurance was rapidly extending coverage to full-time salaried workers in large firms and their families, there was no coverage for the medical costs of the unemployed poor, for workers in low-paying jobs, and the elderly. In this respect the United States differed from most other advanced countries. Johnson wanted the federal government to help with this problem, but the American Medical Association (AMA), still a potent political force at that time, was—as always—deeply suspicious of all government-sponsored health care. Only after Congress had passed two amendments to the Social Security Act that established the Medicare and Medicaid programs, and Johnson had promised that government would not interfere in any way with medical practice and would simply undertake to pay "usual and customary" fees, did the AMA's opposition soften.

The Medicare program covered most of the costs of medical care for the elderly (over age sixty-five) and for some disabled patients, while Medicaid provided insurance for the most vulnerable segments of the indigent and unemployed population. This legislation resulted in a sudden, major expansion of health insurance, covering in particular those citizens who had been least able to pay for their care and therefore were most dependent on the charity of physicians and private community hospitals. Overnight, the federal government became the largest single insurer of health care and relieved physicians and hospitals of the burden of treating many patients who previously could not pay their bills.

Medicare Part A covers a limited number of days of care in hospitals, chronic care facilities, and at home, and it is financed by mandatory payroll taxes. Medicare Part B covers physicians' services and most outpatient medical expenses except prescription drugs; unlike Part A, it is voluntary and is financed in part by general tax revenues, by premiums deducted from Social Security payments, and by co-payments from patients as they receive services. At first, payment for services were, as promised by Johnson, based on "usual and customary" charges, and there was no attempt by government to influence medical decisions. The hostility of the AMA soon waned when it became clear that Medicare Part B was a bonanza for physicians. It gave them expanded scope for treating the elderly, and it greatly enhanced their professional incomes. But later on, some of the good feeling among medical practitioners dissipated, as the cost to the federal government mounted rapidly and the Medicare program tried to contain its expenses by reducing physicians' fees (see Chapter 2).

Medicaid provided federal funds to states on a cost-sharing basis, related inversely to each state's per capita income, and it covered physicians' services, inpatient and outpatient hospital care, long-term nursing facility care, and laboratory and X-ray services. Each state decided on its participation in Medicaid and on the income levels that qualified beneficiaries for coverage. States were also allowed wide latitude in negotiating payments to providers and deciding on the type of insurance they provided.

With the implementation of Medicare and Medicaid in 1966, along with rapidly expanding employment-based private coverage in the 1950s and 1960s, the majority of U.S. citizens had an outside source (a "third party") to pay for most of their medical bills (the first two "parties" are the patient and the provider). This rapid increase in private and public insurance coverage was a powerful stimulus for the growth of medical expenditures, particularly because most of the payment to providers was on a fee-for-service basis, no questions asked.

New specialists, using new procedures and tests and new forms of treatment, could offer patients a level of medical service hardly imaginable only a few decades earlier, and fee-for-service reimbursement from insurance provided the economic incentive to do so. Patients with acute or chronic medical problems were eager to get this high-technology specialty care, particularly since most of the charges were paid by their insurance. Hospitals, where much of the new technology was being deployed, were no less eager to provide it—so long as they could be assured of payment on a "customary" basis, thus guaranteeing a profit. The introduction of new technology in the hands of specialists, expanded insurance coverage, and unregulated fee-for-service payments all combined to rapidly increase the flow of money into the health care system, and thus sowed the seeds of a new, profit-driven industry.

## The Rise of the "Medical-Industrial Complex"

In response to the business opportunities afforded by the abundant new supply of insurance money, a multitude of investor-owned health care facilities appeared in the late 1960s and early 1970s. The first of these were chains of proprietary hospitals, followed by nursing homes and for-profit companies providing home care, laboratory, and imaging services. It was easy to make profits by getting doctors to refer insured patients to these facilities and then charging "customary" rates. For-profit diagnostic facilities, such as clinical laboratories and radiology ("imaging") centers, offered practicing physicians an opportunity to purchase equity interest in exchange for agreements to refer patients. Physicians were also given financial incentives (interest-free loans, discounted office rent, and so on) to admit patients to investor-owned hospitals for diagnosis and treatment and to keep them there as long as deemed not only medically but financially desirable. Proprietary hospitals encouraged physicians who used their facilities to order tests and procedures—with the knowledge that insurance would pay the bills.[10] Some hospitals set up young physicians in private practices located in nearby offices and guaranteed their initial income, with the understanding that their patients would be referred to the sponsoring hospital. Many not-for-profit hospitals, feeling the competition for patients and medical staff from investor-owned hospitals in their communities, followed suit by using some of the same tactics. They, too, became income maximizers and hired practicing physicians to work with them in a medical care system that gradually began to resemble a marketplace more than a social service provided by the community. Although some of the methods hospitals and ambulatory facilities used to increase referrals from practicing physicians were later abandoned because they were ineffective (or illegal), the entrepreneurial drive that infected all facilities has not lessened. Today, medical facilities of all kinds, for-profit and not-for-profit alike, advertise their services heavily—a phenomenon frowned upon and virtually unknown twenty-five or thirty years ago.

Heavy promotion of services, physicians, and facilities, which had formerly been considered unethical, became customary, as both not-for-profit and for-profit providers joined in the competition to expand their markets and increase their income. Competition for patients is not usually based on price. As Arrow had observed in 1963, medical services are largely price-insensitive. Few patients would shop for a low-priced brain surgeon or a hospital with a cut-rate intensive care unit—and certainly not if they were insured. The prices paid for insured services, whether set by providers or insurers, are of little concern to patients as long as they have insurance to pay the bill. In fact, insured patients are often glad to know they have a high-priced medical provider because that suggests high quality. Those relatively few patients who are not insured and pay out of pocket have to pay pretty much whatever providers ask. Competition for patients tends to increase services and therefore increase expenditures on health care.

In 1980, in the *New England Journal of Medicine*, I called attention to the changing, increasingly commercialized face of U.S. medical care, calling it the "new medical-industrial complex."[11] The term was derived from the language used by Dwight D. Eisenhower in his farewell address as president on January 17, 1961, when he warned the nation to beware "the military-industrial complex," a huge armaments industry that had acquired great political and economic power and had begun to influence public policy in matters of national defense. In analogous fashion, I described the rise of a new investor-owned industry that was providing health care services for profit and might reshape the behavior of almost all other health care providers and the system itself. Like the arms industry, this new health care industry could use its powerful lobbying muscle to influence public policies.

I believe this article was the first description and analysis of the commercialization of U.S. medical services that had begun to take shape in the late 1960s. The article's facts were not challenged, but my speculation about the cause of commercialization and its effect on the future of our health care system and on the professional values of physicians had a mixed reception. Some critics agreed with me, but others thought that my concerns were exaggerated or that commercialization should be welcomed as a movement toward better cost control and efficiency, and a more patient-friendly system. In any case, the article was followed by a growing literature on the subject, including many empirical studies. In 1986, the Institute of Medicine of the National Academy of Sciences published a report called "For-Profit Enterprise in Health Care," which carried the inquiry much further, with a particular focus on for-profit hospitals,[12] the findings of which are covered in Chapter 2.

In 1991, I explored this subject again by reviewing the developments since my 1980 article.[13] I reported that the initial explosion of corporate for-profit hospital chains had slowed considerably. In 1980, when I wrote the first piece, there had been approximately

1,000 investor-owned hospitals, which had been increasing at a rate that would have predicted at least a doubling in another decade. Instead, ten years later there were barely 1,400 such hospitals (of a total of 5,000 licensed U.S. hospitals) and the number of corporate chains was no longer increasing. This unexpected slowdown in the net transfer of hospitals to investor ownership was due to constraints on hospital reimbursement by government and private insurers and to increasing local resistance to the corporate takeover of community hospitals (more about that in Chapter 3).

However, investor ownership of medical care facilities had continued to grow. Without the attractions of further investment in acute-care hospital chains, investors turned to other sectors of the health care system. By 1991, proprietary psychiatric hospitals and all kinds of investor-owned outpatient facilities had multiplied because they were not constrained by the government payment regulations that had been applied to general hospitals. Many physicians were among the investors in outpatient facilities, a trend stimulated by a series of U.S. Supreme Court decisions that in effect struck down some of the traditional distinctions between professions and businesses.

## The Courts Apply Antitrust Law to Medicine

In 1943, antitrust laws were first applied to medicine, when the Supreme Court found that the AMA and the Medical Society of the District of Columbia had violated antitrust law by conspiring to "obstruct and restrain" the "business" of Group Health, a prepaid group practice in Washington, D.C.[14] The medical societies had tried to discourage physicians from working for Group Health by denying them membership. The Court sidestepped the question of whether medical practitioners were businesspeople subject to antitrust laws or professionals exempt from such laws by deciding that Group Health was in business and the defendants had interfered with Group Health's freedom to compete for patients. But in 1975, the Court struck a much more direct blow against the notion that medical professionals should enjoy any antitrust immunity. In that year, the Court ruled that the Virginia Bar Association had violated antitrust law by attempting to control legal fees. More generally, this decision[15] found that professional bar organizations were not exempt from antitrust laws, and the ruling extended by implication to such medical professional organizations as the AMA. A series of subsequent court decisions over the next few years seemed to establish the principle that medical societies and physicians enjoyed no blanket professional exemption from antitrust law.[16] Medical organizations such as the AMA, by nature cautious, were no longer willing to set ethical standards that might be seen as limiting business competition.

The Federal Trade Commission believed that these decisions empowered it to ensure that price competition, marketing, advertising, and other kinds of competitive market behavior be encouraged in the health care system. The rationale was that competition in medical care, as with most other goods and services sold in the market, would lower prices and improve quality.[17] However, there is little or no empirical evidence that competition in the delivery of medical care has had any such broad or sustained effect. Nevertheless, the abrupt turnaround in AMA and state medical society policy that followed these court decisions has made it quite clear that fear of antitrust law has tied the hands of professional associations in promulgating and enforcing ethical standards that are threatened when physicians in practice become too caught up in commerce and the pursuit of profitable business deals.

In my view, the application of antitrust law to medicine should be revisited in the courts or Congress. No antitrust law specifically states that the practice of medicine is included in the definition of "interstate commerce"—which is the usual target of such legislation. I think it is debatable whether the public interest is really furthered by always treating it as if it were ordinary commerce. Chief Justice Warren Burger raised this question in his oft-quoted footnote to the opinion he wrote in the 1975 Virginia Bar Association case,[18] and no high court action since then has specifically addressed that issue. The role of antitrust law in medical care would certainly need to be reconsidered if our system were to be redesigned as suggested in Chapter 5. The argument of this book is that the public interest would be better served by a noncommercial approach that restored medical care to a professional service. In a reformed and decommercialized health care system, legal concerns about boycotts, price fixing, and other types of anti-competitive activity would be much less relevant and there would be little or no need for regulation by antitrust law. However, I do believe that medical care should be regulated in other ways, both internally (professionally) and by other kinds of federal and state law.

## Today's Medical Marketplace

There can be little doubt that today's health care system has become thoroughly saturated with market ideology. The majority of private insurance plans are investor owned. About 20 percent of all nongovernmental hospitals are investor owned, including the great majority of psychiatric and specialty hospitals. Responding to the competition for patients, not-for-profit hospitals have taken on many of the attributes of their investor-owned competitors, including the drive to expand their market share and eliminate nonprofitable services—thus making the behavior of for-profit and not-for-profit hospitals increasingly indistinguishable. Almost all private, not-for-profit hospitals are now managed like businesses. They advertise and market their services and exert every effort to fill their beds with insured, paying patients.

In recent years a particularly problematic kind of entrepreneurial hospital has appeared in the United States that specializes in only one kind of highly profitable service, such as orthopedic or cardiovascular surgery, gynecologic surgery, or cancer treatment. They provide little or no treatment to the uninsured, and they are all for-profit, investor-owned businesses. There is no good evidence that their services are more efficient or of better quality than those provided by competing general hospitals. Critics say that they tend to skim off the easiest and most profitable cases, thus threatening the viability of other hospitals in the community that are left to deal with the complicated or indigent patients. But this criticism has not so far been able to stop the trend. These specialty hospitals are rapidly increasing and, at present writing, number about 130.[19] Their growth is primarily the result of support by the specialist physicians who use and invest in them, and of lobbying by the business interests that provide most of the capital.

There has been a large shift in recent years from inpatient to outpatient care as hospital reimbursements have become increasingly regulated. The majority of the numerous freestanding private outpatient facilities are investor owned, including ambulatory surgical centers, diagnostic laboratories, walk-in primary care clinics, imaging centers offering CT scans, MRI, and other advanced methods, and kidney dialysis facilities. Likewise, the majority of nursing homes are investor owned. Special nursing services, including case management services and home health care, are also heavily commercialized.

It is hard to estimate the number of private health care facilities that are now investor owned, but it must be very large. There are no reliable data on this point. My best guess is that at least 40 percent of what is spent on personal health care now goes to investor-owned organizations and facilities that provide those services.[20] Whatever the exact size of the investor-owned health care system, it is certainly large enough to have drastically changed the behavior of most institutions (for-profit or not), as well as the behavior and attitudes of almost all physicians.

Many physicians have invested in for-profit health care facilities and services or are themselves incorporated as for-profit organizations to deliver specialized services. Almost all of the specialty hospitals and most of the outpatient surgery centers are either owned by physicians or have physicians as important investors. After the AMA dropped its injunctions against advertising because of concern about antitrust liability, many physicians began to advertise and market their services, and in some specialties they began to sell health care products (such as skin care preparations and nutritional supplements) in their offices. They also began to make profitable deals with manufacturers of the drugs, medical goods, appliances, and prostheses they use and prescribe. In short, the commercialization of the health care system has now extended to individual physicians and in many cases has been actively aided and abetted by them. Physicians are supposed to be fiduciaries for their patients, so financial ties to the facilities and technology that they use for their patients create an obvious conflict of interest. Although there are some legal constraints that limit physician investment in health care facilities, there are many loopholes that allow much of this investment to continue. However, few laws prohibit the innumerable financial arrangements that doctors may make with pharmaceutical companies and manufacturers of medical devices. These conflicts of interest now pervade the practice of medicine, and they inevitably increase medical expenditures because they encourage physicians to use the facilities, procedures, tests, drugs, and medical devices in which they have a financial interest, without sufficient consideration of costs and benefits or the availability of alternatives that may be less expensive and just as good or better.[21]

For example, I recently learned about a company that markets an expensive patented device (list price $149,000) that can be used in the doctor's office for the treatment of back pain. Physicians can buy or lease these devices and, according to the company's ads, can increase their practice income by several hundred thousand dollars a year. Under the lease arrangement, the company will install and service the device without charge in exchange for a per-treatment fee from the doctor, who can then charge the patient's medical insurance enough to make a substantial profit. The company recommends a series of twenty or thirty treatments for each patient, which can be administered by a company-trained office assistant (allowing the physician to continue seeing other patients). It recommends a fee of $5,000–$7,000 for each patient so treated. The company also provides marketing advice and materials designed to recruit new patients and generate referrals from other doctors. The device itself is approved by the Food and Drug Administration (FDA) as "safe and effective" but has not yet been systematically compared with the many other techniques for the treatment of back pain. Neither is there any good evidence on the duration of the benefit afforded by this device.

Here, then, is an arrangement in which the company and the physician are in effect business partners in promoting the use of an expensive medical device that has not yet been adequately evaluated. The company's advertising materials, which I studied carefully, emphasize the financial benefits to physicians at least as much as the alleged (but still unproven) benefits to patients. Testimonials abound in the company's advertising material, but carefully controlled clinical studies with adequate follow-up results in peer-reviewed medical journals are not to be found. Is this an example of medical progress or medical entrepreneurialism—or both? Does this device save money by avoiding surgery, or does it simply add to the expense of health care? In the absence of reliable scientific information about clinical benefits, it is hard to be sure there has been any medical progress. What does seem clear, however, is that the very substantial financial benefits to the physician are far beyond the time or professional expertise required in using the machine. It certainly looks more like a profitable business opportunity for the company and the doctor than the professional practice of medicine. Furthermore, physicians who choose to use these devices would very likely have a high opinion of their effectiveness and would not be inclined to consider other types of treatment. Unfortunately, these problems are typical of the innumerable deals physicians are now making with health care businesses.

I am puzzled that the consequences of this sort of commercial transformation of medical care have so far generated relatively little concern among health policy experts. A few authors have written about this change, but virtually no connections have been made between it and the current problems of our health care system. Health policy articles often consider whether we should rely largely on market forces or on government regulation to control health care costs and whether private insurance should be based on employment or individual ownership. But there is little discussion of the social and health effects of the growth of investor ownership and the transformation of health care into a gigantic profit-oriented business. I suspect this has something to do with the general view that American society should depend primarily on private business, not government, and that private entrepreneurship is an essential part of American culture.

To most economists and businesspeople, it probably seems perfectly natural that health care should be sold like a commercial service by profit-seeking firms, despite the fact that until the late 1960s, there was neither organized private investment in the delivery of health care, nor large publicly traded for-profit health care corporations. Those who believe medical care is simply another service being sold in another market see no reason why it shouldn't be distributed and marketed by for-profit businesses, or why physicians shouldn't have financial interests in the products and facilities they use in caring for patients. They believe physicians, who have always sold their services, are in essence profit-making vendors, constrained perhaps by certain professional norms, but vendors nevertheless. What might seem surprising to these observers is not that so many health care facilities are owned by for-profit businesses and so many physicians have entrepreneurial interests, but that not-for-profit private facilities and non-entrepreneurial private practitioners still exist at all. In their view, physicians and medical care facilities are simply acting as economically rational entities, lawfully and naturally responding to market incentives.

I don't wish to be misunderstood about the practice of medicine. I am not saying that business considerations were never a part of the medical profession before the commercial tsunami of the 1970s and 1980s, or that physicians were in the past unconcerned about their income. In the minds of physicians, business concerns have always been intermingled with the social and ethical obligations of medical care. The practice of medicine has always had its entrepreneurs, and practitioners have always paid attention to earning their living. In this respect, physicians have been no different from those pursuing careers in other professions, such as law, education, architecture, and science. But the commitment to serve patients' medical needs (as well as the needs of public health) and the special nature of the relation between doctor and patient placed a particularly heavy professional obligation on physicians that was expected to supersede considerations of personal gain—and usually did. A similar commitment also motivated the modestly salaried managers and the volunteer trustees of the community-oriented, non-entrepreneurial facilities that typified private hospitals until just a few decades ago.

With new financial opportunities and the onslaught of investor-owned health care, the commitment to social service has been overtaken by an entrepreneurial imperative. Most private hospitals, whether investor-owned or not, now behave like profit-seeking, market-share-seeking businesses, and they are increasingly managed by high-paid corporate-style executives whose attention is fixed on the bottom line. Even many teaching hospitals and academic health centers are now engaged in entrepreneurial activities that are hardly compatible with their primary professional commitments. Doctors are succumbing to the same business incentives. Competition for patients, resulting from the higher ratio of doctors to population, probably also makes today's physicians more interested in generating additional income from entrepreneurial arrangements. Gradually over the past few decades, health care has come to resemble a vast profit-oriented industry.

This new climate has been reflected in the shifting policies of the AMA. During the many years before, and in the first few decades after World War II, when it represented the views of the great majority of doctors, the AMA not only defended the economic interests of its members but also tried to protect the health and medical welfare of the public. Notwithstanding its vigilant defense of physicians' interests, it insisted that doctors were not engaged in trade and were bound by professional norms that placed patients' interests first. Physicians were therefore enjoined to avoid advertising and self-promotion, and were expected to limit their professional income to reasonable returns from the care of their patients. The AMA also believed that corporations should not be responsible for the delivery of medical care, because the "corporate practice of medicine" was not compatible with the requirements of a professional relation between doctors and their patients.[22]

Although the AMA still vigorously supports "professionalism" and a primary commitment to patients, most of its former injunctions against commercial activities by physicians and the "corporate practice of medicine" have disappeared in response to the courts' interpretation of antitrust law. Having been found guilty of limiting competition by restricting the business activities of physicians, the AMA changed its guidelines to allow doctors to engage in most kinds of commercial activity and entrepreneurialism, so long as they are legal, disclosed to patients, and (in each physician's judgment) not prejudicial to the best interests of their patients.[23] Indeed, many publications for physicians, from the AMA and other medical professional organizations, now regularly provide information about "the doctor's business" and advise physicians on how they can enhance the profitability of their practice by adopting business techniques. It seems clear that, on the advice of its lawyers, the AMA has decided not to appeal the antitrust decisions that have in effect blurred much of the distinction between commerce and medical care.

A growing number of medical schools offer joint programs leading to combined M.D.-M.B.A. degrees, and business school professors have joined economists in prescribing health care policies.[24] In short, business and medical practice are no longer generally considered to be at odds—this, despite the inescapable fact that the essential nature of the relation between doctor and patient is quite different from that between vendors and consumers in commercial markets.

Whatever the AMA's resistance to the emergence of the medical marketplace might have been in the past, it has been weakened by more than court decisions and the financial realities of the "medical-industrial complex." The AMA is no longer the powerful voice of America's physicians that it once was. Its influence has greatly declined over the past few decades, as an increasing number of specialty organizations have claimed the primary allegiance of most of the new specialists. In addition, many physicians have reservations about the AMA's political and business policies. Currently, fewer than one-third of practicing physicians are members, barely half the percentage of a few decades ago.

## Why Aren't Other Countries So Commercialized?
## A Short Answer

Why didn't the health care systems of other advanced countries, which experienced to a varying degree the same expansion, specialization, and technical development as the United States, follow our example in becoming highly privatized and commercialized? Suffice it to say here that these other countries (for example, the United Kingdom, Germany, France, and Sweden) had universal, publicly supervised health insurance systems in place before, or soon after, the postwar technological revolution in medical care began. Unlike the fragmented and decentralized U.S. system, these public plans prohibit or discourage private enterprise from gaining more than a marginal position in their health care systems, and they usually regulate the prices paid to doctors and hospitals. The strong incentives to commercialization that were unopposed in the United States were essentially blocked by the prior existence of national health programs in these countries.

Furthermore, the citizens of most other technically advanced, democratic countries have a different attitude toward the role of government in assuring health care for all. In the United States, there is widespread suspicion of government involvement in private affairs (such as health care), which doesn't exist to nearly the same degree elsewhere. Social solidarity and government protection of individual welfare are accepted values in most developed countries. It has been only recently that the rising cost of modern health care everywhere and the sales pitch of an increasingly globalized "medical-industrial complex" have been tempting other countries to follow us down the garden path of commercialized medical services.

# 2

## THE CONSEQUENCES OF COMMERCIALIZED CARE

For the love of money is the root of all evil.

—1 TIMOTHY 6:10 (KING JAMES VERSION)

Few trends could so thoroughly undermine the very foundations of our free society as the acceptance by corporate officials of a social responsibility other than to make as much money for their stockholders as possible.

—MILTON FRIEDMAN,
*CAPITALISM AND FREEDOM*, 1962

LET'S FIRST LOOK AT THE RAPID GROWTH IN MEDICAL EXPENDITURES that accompanied the events described in the previous chapter. To call this relentless rise in costs an "explosion" may be a little hyperbolic, but it certainly has had striking effects on the health care system and on our national economy. *Cost is the central problem in health care* and it generates or aggravates most of the other problems in the system. Therefore, controlling health costs is the essential first step to providing better health care to more people. It is also a prerequisite for allowing us to allocate sufficient public resources to education, Social Security, maintenance of public works, national security, law enforcement, and all the other essential functions of government.

A useful way to measure health care expenditures is to express them as a percentage of the gross domestic product (GDP), which corrects for the growth of the total economy and includes the effects of increased population and inflation in general prices. Starting with the end of World War II, this measure at first rose relatively slowly. Health care accounted for about 4 percent of the GDP in 1950 and about 5.5 percent in 1966, the year Medicare and Medicaid went into effect.

Figure 1[1] shows the trends in health care expenditures, expressed as a percent of the GDP, beginning in 1960 and ending in 2004 (vertical line). Projected spending is extended to 2014. Trend lines are shown separately for Medicare spending; all public spending, including Medicare, Medicaid, federal employees, and veterans; all private spending, including employment-based and out-of-pocket spending; and total health spending. The figure shows only the actual disbursements of money for health care. It does not include the calculated cost to the federal government of the tax revenues not collected on the health care benefits paid to workers by their employers, which are by law specifically exempt from taxation.

For the first half of the 1960s, expenditures in both the private and the public sectors continued to rise at the slow rate characteristic of the previous decade. Then public expenditures suddenly began to increase more rapidly. This increase was due primarily to the appearance of Medicare and Medicaid insurance, which for a time caused the growth of public expenditures to outpace that of private expenditures. Except for transient slowdowns in the mid-1980s and 1990s, all health expenditures have continued to rise ever since. However, as shown by the dashed and dotted lines in the figure, public spending has generally increased more rapidly than private spending. At first, private spending greatly exceeded all public expenditures, but the difference between the two has narrowed progressively. They are nearly equal now, and if the calculated loss of tax revenues were included, public expenditures would exceed those in the private sector.

43

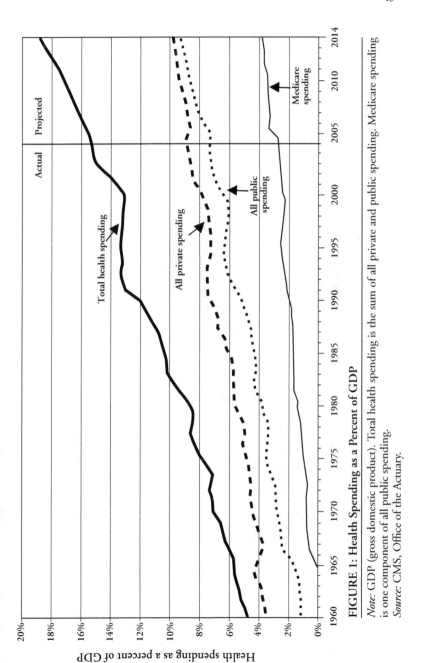

FIGURE 1: Health Spending as a Percent of GDP

*Note:* GDP (gross domestic product). Total health spending is the sum of all private and public spending. Medicare spending is one component of all public spending.
*Source:* CMS, Office of the Actuary.

In 2005, total expenditures were estimated to be well over $2 trillion, more than 16 percent of the GDP, or on average about $7,000 for every resident of the United States—young or old, healthy or sick.

The average rate of increase in health expenditures since the late 1960s has been between 9 and 10 percent per year, which is more than twice the rate of general price inflation. The National Health Statistics Group at the Centers for Medicare and Medicaid Services has recently predicted that health expenditures will continue to rise at an average annual rate of over 7 percent for the next decade. This government agency believes that by the year 2015, the United States will be spending more than $4 trillion, or about 20 percent of the GDP.

Most experts believe that a major part of the inflation-adjusted increase in medical expenditures is accounted for by the delivery of ever-greater quantities of complicated and expensive services per capita, which is another way of saying that increased use of new technology drives the cost explosion.[2] Examples of this expensive "new technology" include cardiovascular interventions such as heart surgery and the use of coronary artery stents and implanted cardiac pacemakers; replacement of arthritic hip and knee joints; transplantation of hearts, kidneys, and livers; improved diagnostic imaging with CAT scans and MRIs; fiberoptic colonoscopy; and the wide use of expensive new prescription drugs. In virtually every specialized field, myriad technical advances have produced new and more expensive devices and techniques for diagnosis and treatment that contribute to the cost of health care. The experts also believe that another major contributor to the continued rise in expenditures is the existence of insurance, which makes patients less reluctant to seek medical services than they otherwise would be.[3] An increase in the average age of the population and in the prevalence of chronic diseases, such as diabetes, arthritis, and Alzheimer's disease, are thought to be much smaller factors.

I find it surprising, however, that in their discussion of the rise in health care expenditures, so few analysts have looked beyond the causes mentioned above to consider the role of physicians—the way they are paid, and the incentives that motivate them in a commercialized market. As Arrow first noted, the market for medical services is not like other markets because of the great influence of physicians in determining what resources will be used in a given situation. When physicians have strong incentives to maximize their income, such as occurs in our commercialized, competitive system, they will increase health expenditures by ordering more tests, procedures, and treatments—particularly if there is open-ended insurance to pay the charges on a piecework, "cost-plus" basis.

Although there is no economic law that determines what percentage of the national economy or of personal expenditures should be spent on health care, it is obvious that the more we spend on health care, the less we can spend on other needs and wants. Relative to all the other components of personal consumption spending in the United States (for instance, food, housing, transportation, recreation, and so on) personal expenditures on health care have been increasing steadily over the past few decades. They now account for the single-largest share of personal consumption (about 19 percent). Total health care spending has been rising at nearly equal rates in both the public and private sectors, and the cost is threatening the fiscal stability of both government and business. Both of these major payers are now struggling to control their costs by reducing their health insurance obligations, and to the extent they do so, the number of uninsured and underinsured citizens increases.

## Has It Been Worth the Money?

Not everyone is seriously worried about these rising costs. Some economists take a more sanguine view, arguing that increased expenditures are buying better health and longer life, and that these benefits are well worth the costs. I know many medical research scientists and leaders in academic medicine who hold similar views about rising expenditures on new clinical technology. What better way is there to spend our resources, they ask, than to develop and use medical technology to extend the human life span, eliminate disease and disability, and improve the quality of life for everyone? There are even some who believe that new technology, based on research, will ultimately reduce medical expenditures by curing or preventing the diseases that have been responsible for rising costs.

Prominent among the economists arguing that the benefits of medical expenditures are worth the costs is Professor David M. Cutler of Harvard University. In a 2004 book and in a subsequent article in the *New England Journal of Medicine*,[4] he used economic methods to estimate the value of the years of life gained by the use of new medical technology and concluded, "On average the increases in medical spending since 1960 have provided reasonable value." Robert E. Hall and Charles I. Jones, professors of economics at Stanford and U.C.–Berkeley, respectively, have recently made a similar argument, but use more formal econometric methodology.[5] They consider why new technologies are developed and used, and they propose an economic model that explains the growth in medical expenditures as a rising evaluation of extended life years by the "consumers" of health care. They speculate that "[a]s people get richer, the most valuable channel for spending is to purchase additional years of life." They predict that "optimal health spending" will rise to more than 30 percent of the GDP by the year 2050, and they think this reflects the free choice of consumers who prefer to spend their money on health rather than on other items of personal consumption.

There are several major flaws in these economic arguments. In the first place, whatever monetary "value" is placed on the medical longevity benefits of health expenditures in the United States (and this "value," in my judgment is purely theoretical because, despite what economists may say, human life is priceless and cannot be assigned a monetary value), the fact remains that other advanced countries produce equal or better benefits to the public's health at much lower cost (see note 8 in this chapter). It simply cannot be argued that we are getting "good value" if the citizens of other countries live longer and enjoy better health than we do, while spending much less in achieving those benefits.

Secondly, underlying the arguments of Cutler and those of Hall and Jones is the implicit but dubious assumption that the recent extension of average life span in this country is largely or entirely the result of increased health care expenditures. But correlation is not the same as causation, and despite the statistical and temporal correlations between increased expenditures on medical technology and the extension of average life span, we know that at least some of our improved health is due to changing social factors such as improved living conditions, education, and a healthier lifestyle. Many gains in public health are independent of technical medical care, so the results of economic analyses of costs and benefits of medical care must be viewed with caution, if not outright skepticism.

Third, this type of economic reasoning seems to assume that health care expenditures result from the accumulated free choices (or "demand") of individual "consumers" who are weighing how they will spend their money. That is far from the case. Out-of-pocket expenditures account for less than one-fourth of total health expenditures; the rest is paid by third parties, usually insurers, who do not personally receive, or benefit from, the care being given. Furthermore, irrespective of who pays, those who receive the care do not make a free choice, like ordinary consumers. They usually receive care because the circumstances of their illness or injury create a need. The identification of that need and the determination of the appropriate response are the responsibility of their physicians. Even when medical services are preventive or elective, they are usually initiated on the advice of a physician, who, in a fee-for-service system, may have financial incentives to provide certain services—particularly expensive high-technology procedures. So if most health care does not represent a voluntary choice by the recipient, and if doctors' financial interests may influence "demand," expenditures on health should not be considered simply a measure of how much of their income consumers wish to devote to this purpose, as Hall and Jones would have us believe. Traditional "supply and demand" forces are usually not operative in the medical care system, and prices are not nearly as important in determining the demand for services as they are in other sectors of the economy.

And finally, no judgment about the benefits purchased by expenditures on health care can overlook the financial pain inflicted by rising costs. There is a huge and growing cohort of Americans who simply cannot afford the costs and are being excluded from the benefits of medical care. At 16 percent of the GDP, rising health costs are threatening the financial stability of government and business. Arguments that our health care benefits are worth the money carry little weight with a federal government that is desperately trying to reduce the rising costs of Medicare or with state governments struggling to contain their Medicaid expenditures. Neither do they satisfy corporations like General Motors (GM) and other U.S. auto manufacturers that are in a life-and-death struggle to control their enormous outlays for the medical care of workers and retirees. It is hard to imagine that government or businesses will allow their costs to go much higher, and it is just as hard to imagine much more cost being shifted to average and low-income citizens.

In short, I think the reassurances of those who find no serious problem with our rising health costs are unrealistic and unpersuasive. Considering that we spend so much more on medical care than any other advanced country, we ought to expect health outcomes at least as good, and our citizens ought to be at least as satisfied with the system. But we can claim neither. The conclusion seems inescapable:

We should not be satisfied with our lavishly expensive system, because we are not getting our money's worth by a long shot. What is more, the problem is likely to get even worse.

## The Role of Commercialization in Increasing Costs

How much of the escalation of health spending can be attributed to the commercial transformation of health care, which began in the mid-1960s, and how much to the many other antecedent and continuing factors such as fee-for-service payment, the proliferation of new technology, the aging of the population, and the growth of insurance? Assuming that these other factors had been in place but the health care system had remained largely not-for-profit and without investor-owned health insurance or health care corporations, would we now be facing the same cost crisis?

That question cannot be decisively answered. However, we do know that investor-owned businesses invariably seek to increase their sales income, and this usually means promotion of increased expenditures on their products. Investor-owned businesses always want to grow and there is no reason businesses in health care should be any different. Businesses are like babies; they must grow to thrive. From this fact alone one can suspect that the delivery of health care services by investor-owned businesses probably has something to do with increasing expenditures on those services.

But this isn't nearly the whole story. The impact of investor-owned businesses on health care expenditures extends beyond the care they directly manage or deliver and involves almost the entire health care system. Investor-owned health care businesses have created a competitive commercialized environment in which the not-for-profit institutions must also survive, and which also offers many incentives to physicians who wish to share in the opportunities for private gain. Competition for income from paying patients has forced the not-for-profit hospitals to behave much like their business competitors, and the lure of business profits has changed far too many physicians from professionally committed caregivers to medical entrepreneurs.

Competition in health care differs from competition in commercial markets in that it does not involve price, so there is no economic benefit to the public. Although hospitals may differ in their charges for similar services, they never advertise themselves as offering the cheapest prices. Physicians don't advertise their fees, either. Instead, competition among health care institutions and physicians is largely a contest to attract well-insured patients and provide profitable services. In this competition, private not-for-profit hospitals behave pretty much like their investor-owned rivals. Many physicians become part of the competition. They join with hospitals in promoting the use of expensive services and technology, or they directly compete with them by owning or leasing diagnostic or therapeutic equipment for use in their offices. A health care system such as ours, in which much less than half of the hospitals are owned by investors and much expensive equipment is found in private offices, thus ends up behaving as if it were almost entirely an income-maximizing for-profit industry. Expenditures inevitably rise.

The relatively high overhead expenses of many business institutions also serve to drive the cost of health care up. Investor-owned hospitals usually spend considerable money on high executive salaries and bonuses, consultants, legal advice, brokers, marketing and advertising, back-office operations, public relations and lobbying, and many other expenses that are common in business but until the arrival of the "medical-industrial complex," were absent in not-for-profit hospitals. These overhead expenses apply as well to investor-owned insurance plans, which spend more money than public insurers and not-for-profit plans on underwriting and avoiding beneficiaries who may need more than average care.

Higher administrative expenses add to the cost of doing business. They also add to the prices charged, because for-profit organizations must earn enough net income to generate profit, attract investors, and increase the value of their stock.

To stay competitive, not-for-profit hospitals have had to take on many of the same overhead expenses. They are usually not driven to earn the same level of net income as the investor-owned hospitals and they are expected to be more responsive to community needs, but all of today's hospitals are much more businesslike than a few decades ago, regardless of whether they are for-profit or not-for-profit. The CEO of any hospital today will confirm that the administrative infrastructure of the institution has become more elaborate and expensive than ever. There are far more business and administrative personnel, far more expenditures for billing and collecting, and far higher executive salaries than ever before in all health care institutions. This increases costs and must ultimately drive up expenditures for hospital care.

## Inequity: Another Result of Commercialization

Inequity—inequality of access to essential health care—is another major problem with our health care system, and without question commercialization of the system has played a large role here as well. Markets are not concerned with justice or equity. When private health care and insurance are sold in commercial markets by profit-driven providers, access is limited largely to those who can afford to pay—or those whose employers pay for them. As expenditures for care continue to rise in both the private and the public sectors, insurance premiums sooner or later must rise with them.

When premiums rise, government and employers, the two main payers of health care, are forced to leave a growing number of people uninsured or underinsured, or to require more co-payments or deductibles from beneficiaries. At present, nearly 47 million people in the United States are without insurance, and many more have only limited coverage. These numbers are rising rapidly as government and employers continue to reduce their benefits and thin out the ranks of the adequately insured. There can be little doubt that the swelling army of uninsured and underinsured, and the progressive fraying of coverage, are the result of the high costs in our market-driven system. This has serious consequences for the health and welfare of many of the uninsured, as recent studies have shown.[6]

Who will now care for the indigent and uninsured sick? Investor-owned health care facilities say that they pay taxes for this purpose and that tax-exempt private facilities or tax-supported government institutions should take the responsibility. But if they are to remain viable, private tax-exempt hospitals often must compete with investor-owned hospitals and ambulatory facilities in the same community. Teaching hospitals (which are the largest tax-exempt private health care institutions) say they are particularly hard pressed because they are not adequately compensated for their educational and research costs, or for the costs of the unprofitable but expensive services they are obliged to maintain as providers of last resort. For these reasons, the large not-for-profit teaching hospitals claim they cannot afford the charity care expected of them any more than can nonteaching, not-for-profit community hospitals. Even though not-for-profit private hospitals still generally provide more unreimbursed care and more unprofitable services than investor-owned hospitals, they have come to resemble the latter in their businesslike interest in maximizing their revenues. Their top management is rewarded, much like the management of investor-owned hospitals, in relation to the net income earned by the hospital.

At the same time, tax-supported government hospitals and clinics are struggling with limited funds and are unable to deal with the increasing burden of unreimbursed care. To compound the problem, there are many large areas that lack tax-supported hospitals. It is an indictment of our health care system and a national disgrace that we have done so little to address this situation, even as it grows worse. We need a new health care system that deals with the maldistribution of community facilities and encourages not-for-profit hospitals of all types to return to their original function of providing health care for their communities, with less emphasis on the bottom line. Teaching hospitals, of course, have additional responsibilities that need special support, and a new system must provide it.

## The Quality of Care

The other major problem with U.S. health care today has to do with its quality. According to many independent studies, and a major report from the Institute of Medicine (IOM) of the National Academy of Sciences,[7] there are very significant deficiencies and variations in the quality of care provided by our health care system. A recent report from The Commonwealth Fund[8] scores the performance of U.S. health care in comparison with other countries or with accepted standards. By most measures, the United States is no better than average and sometimes worse. I believe these deficiencies in quality are a consequence of the commercialization and fragmentation of our system. When health care is provided largely by solo physicians and by independent hospital and ambulatory facilities, all competing for "market share" and interested primarily in promoting their own services, one cannot expect optimal or even uniform quality of care, regardless of whether the facilities are investor owned or not-for-profit.

Unlike its effect in most commercial markets, competition for income in health care is more likely to harm the quality of service than to improve it. Large variations in quality, fragmentation and narrow specialization of services, failure of much of the system to meet basic standards of care, and a high incidence of medical error are predictable when market forces rather than professional norms control the delivery system. Lacking consumers who can independently judge the quality of service and make informed choices about spending their own money, market-driven health care is not effectively guided by its customers. However, health care consumers, particularly well-insured consumers of elective care, are often attracted by fancy amenities and luxuries that have nothing to do with the quality of medical care but increase its costs. Without sufficient government regulation, market-driven care is not compelled to meet society's needs. Often lacking oversight by unbiased physicians, the market cannot always be relied upon to meet the medical needs of patients. On the other hand, market-driven health care does have strong incentives that encourage aggressive advertising and self-serving, "profits-first" policies among its providers.[9]

The IOM report on quality of care, which was mentioned above, calls for many changes in the way medical care is provided, including adoption of a uniform, integrated electronic-record system and integration of medical services through more teamwork between different specialists and facilities. But these changes are virtually impossible in a health care system dominated by market forces, because they would require cooperation, not competition, among all the providers of a patient's care. This is best achieved by a reorganization of the medical care system such as will be proposed in Chapter 5, which recommends that teams of physicians practice in prepaid multi-specialty groups.

### The Empirical Evidence

I have been arguing that commercialization of health care services has spurred a rapidly increasing growth in health expenditures over the past four decades and has exacerbated the problems of access and quality that now plague the system. I believe these arguments are logical and consistent with the history of U.S. health care, but I acknowledge that objective, quantitative evidence showing the superiority of not-for-profit facilities over investor-owned facilities would strengthen my case. Turning now to a consideration of such evidence, I will also note that such comparisons are difficult and fraught with pitfalls that could bias the results. I have tried to select for discussion the best studies—those published in reputable, peer-reviewed professional journals by authors without financial conflicts of interest. I begin with a landmark report from the Institute of Medicine of the National Academy of Sciences.

## The Institute of Medicine Report

In 1986, the IOM published a report titled "For-Profit Enterprise in Health Care,"[10] which critically examined the then-existing literature in this field, with particular emphasis on hospitals. I was one of the twenty-two members of the committee that conducted this study. The committee included experts in almost all the relevant professional disciplines, as well as three representatives of the for-profit health care industry. The report focused on the most reliable, published comparisons of the behavior of hospitals in investor-owned chains with that of their not-for-profit counterparts. I will quote only a few of its salient conclusions.

With respect to *charges to payers*: "The committee found that the rise in investor ownership of hospitals has increased health care costs to payers . . . by an amount averaging 8 to 24 percent per admission, depending on the method of payment." "On a per-day basis, charges range up to 29 percent higher in investor-owned hospitals."[11]

Concerning *hospital operating expenses*: "Studies generally show higher per-case expenses in investor-owned hospitals, but the differences are not always statistically significant."[12] Although standard economic theory predicts greater efficiency in for-profit than in not-for-profit organizations, the expected ability of investor-owned for-profit organizations to produce the same services at lower cost than their not-for-profit counterparts was not demonstrated.

With regard to the effect of for-profit hospitals on *access to care* by patients who cannot afford to pay, the results were clear: "[F]or-profit hospitals proportionately provide less uncompensated care than do not-for-profit hospitals, although there are substantial variations in the magnitude of this difference."[13] In some states with large numbers of for-profit hospitals (for example, Florida, Texas, Tennessee, and Virginia), the differences in the percent of uncompensated care between the two classes of hospitals were highest, sometimes twofold. Because in private hospitals, regardless of ownership, only a relatively small percent of patients do not pay, the absolute differences between investor-owned and not-for-profit private hospitals were only a few percentage points, but this translates nationwide into large numbers of patients.

The committee noted that available measures of hospital *quality* at that time were too insensitive and too few to permit any definite conclusions about differences in quality of care between for-profit and not-for-profit hospitals and so withheld its judgment.

The committee concluded that "available evidence on differences between for-profit and not-for-profit health care organizations is not sufficient to justify a recommendation that investor ownership of health care organizations be either opposed or supported by public policy." It added, *"However, the for-profit mode cannot now be seen as a possible solution to such important public policy issues as control of health care costs, ensuring access to care, or maintaining quality of care"* (italics mine).[14]

Seven of the committee members (I among them) felt compelled to add a "supplementary statement" at the end of the report, saying that *"we are concerned about what would happen if for-profit institutions assumed a dominant role in our health care system* (italics mine). . . . A substantial increase in the for-profit sector's share of the health system could: (1) Put further pressure on hospitals, voluntary organizations and other facilities that provide needed but less profitable services; (2) Create powerful centers of influence to affect public policy; and (3) Increase the drift of the health care system toward com-

mercialism and away from medicine's service orientation." These
seven members (a lawyer, two sociologists, a philosopher, a consumer-
advocate, and two physicians) concluded their statement with:
"These concerns reinforce the implication of the committee's report
that *we would have little to gain and possibly much to lose, if for-profit
corporations came to dominate our health care system*" (italics mine).[15]

That was 1986, and since then, although investor-owned chain
hospitals did not continue their rapid multiplication, many other
kinds of investor-owned health care businesses delivering care outside
the hospital (where most of the rise in expenditures has occurred) did
increase. Even if these businesses do not now constitute the majority
of the organizations in our health care system (although they certainly
do in some parts of it), they are numerous and influential enough to
have changed the behavior of the whole system and the physicians
who work in it. In effect, for-profit corporations now "dominate" our
health care system, as my IOM colleagues and I feared. We now also
have more comparative data by which to judge the effects of this
domination, and they clearly justify our earlier concerns.

## Empirical Studies Since the IOM Report

Let's now look more closely at some of the best and most significant studies published since the 1986 IOM report.

### *Hospital Costs and Expenditures on Hospital Care*

I have not seen any additional carefully controlled direct comparisons of charges by for-profit and not-for-profit hospitals, but there
have been a number of studies revealing other significant differences.
An interesting report in 1999 compared Medicare spending in geographic areas in which all acute-care hospitals were for-profit with
spending in areas in which all the hospitals were not-for-profit.[16]

Adjusted mean per capita Medicare spending on inpatient care, as well as total spending, was much higher in the for-profit areas, and spending rose when all not-for-profit hospitals in an area were converted to for-profit ownership.

In a 1997 study covering all acute-care hospitals, total hospital expenses per admission (not the same as charges to patients) were found to be almost 10 percent higher in for-profit hospitals.[17] Most of this difference was due to higher administrative costs in the for-profits, where administration accounted for 34 percent of total hospital costs, as compared with 25 percent of total costs attributed to administration in the not-for-profit hospitals. On the other hand, for-profit hospitals spent less money on professional in-house clinical personnel (such as nurses and staff physicians), which might have something to do with differences in the quality of care.

### The Quality of Hospital Care

The quality of hospital care, particularly in general acute-care hospitals that admit a wide variety of acutely and chronically ill adults, is hard to measure. However, one careful study in 2002[18] reviewed all the available published data from U.S. private for-profit and not-for-profit hospitals, pooled the results, and found that the risk of patient death was 2 percent higher in the for-profit hospitals. The large numbers of hospitals studied, and the care with which the authors controlled for other factors that could have influenced the outcome, give these results more clinical and statistical significance than might at first appear from this relatively small difference. Since there is no reason to believe physicians caring for patients in for-profit hospitals are on average less competent than physicians in not-for-profit hospitals (indeed, in a given community they are often the same individuals), I am inclined to attribute any difference in mortality risk to reduced staffing with doctors and nurses at the investor-owned hospitals, as reported in the 1997 study mentioned above.

Another telling comparison of not-for-profit and investor-owned hospitals was recently published[19] in which the types of medical services provided by the two groups of institutions were examined. The results clearly showed that investor-owned hospitals were more likely to offer profitable services (for instance, cardiac catheterization, women's health care, cardiac surgery, pediatric intensive care) and less likely to offer relatively unprofitable services (for example, HIV/AIDS care, trauma treatment, drug addiction outpatient services, psychiatry emergency services) than private not-for-profit hospitals serving similar populations.

Economists might say that such behavior is entirely "rational," because the investor-owned hospitals are responding appropriately to market incentives. But what may be economically "rational" may be very bad social policy for the communities these hospitals are supposed to serve. Many of the unprofitable services are needed by the communities, which expect their private hospitals to cross-subsidize money-losing services with profits earned from other services. When investor-owned hospitals fail to do that, health care in the communities they serve may suffer. And if, as I have already suggested, not-for-profit hospitals also allow competitive financial pressures to influence their own decisions about what kinds of services to provide, then the whole health care system can be affected.

### Kidney Dialysis Units

Comparisons of the quality of care in investor-owned kidney dialysis units versus not-for-profit facilities are consistent with the report of increased mortality in for-profit hospitals. The most convincing of these comparisons is a study published in 1999 of clinical outcomes in dialysis units, involving patients with end-stage renal disease who began their treatment in 1990 to 1993.[20] These patients were followed for three to six years, unless they died before then or they were placed on a waiting list for a kidney transplant.

At the time of this study, over 200,000 patients of all ages with kidney failure were being treated in this country, at a total cost of approximately 13 billion dollars. Costs are largely funded by Medicare, as established in 1972 through amendments to the Social Security law. Medicare pays all dialysis units the same comprehensive fee, per patient treated, and that must cover all the costs, regardless of the service provided and the resources used. The only exception is the cost of injectable drugs, for example, erythropoietin (EPO) for anemia, which is separately reimbursed by Medicare. More than two-thirds of all dialysis units were then (and still are) owned by investors. To make a profit for their owners, investor-owned units must run at or near capacity and keep their expenses down. Expenses are determined by such things as the number and training level of nursing and technical staff, the duration of each dialysis treatment, and whether dialysis equipment is used more than once. All of these factors can also influence patient survival, so when dialysis units reduce their expenses by cutting corners on such things, they may jeopardize the welfare of their patients, although that, of course, is not their intention.

When appropriate adjustments are made for the characteristics of the patients being treated (including the diseases responsible for the kidney failure, and the age of patients), one very clear indication of the quality of dialysis treatment is average length of survival. Transplantation of a healthy kidney to replace a patient's diseased kidneys is generally considered to be better treatment than dialysis, and kidney specialists think most patients on dialysis should receive a transplant as soon as a suitable donor can be found. Therefore, another measure of the quality of care given by dialysis centers is the number of patients they refer for transplantation. But a dialysis patient who receives a transplant leaves the dialysis unit, so there are business incentives for the physicians caring for the patients in the for-profit facility (who often are also investors or owners) to be a little less aggressive in recommending this treatment and getting their patients on a waiting list for transplantation.

In this study, clearly the best of its kind to that time, investigators discovered, after adjusting their data for differences in sociodemographic and clinical characteristics of patients and for certain characteristics of the dialysis centers themselves, that *the mortality rate was 20 percent higher, and the likelihood of being placed on a waiting list for transplantation 26 percent lower, in the for-profit facilities.* They did not have data on the net income of the investor-owned and not-for-profit units or on expenditures for the various factors mentioned that contribute both to expenses and possibly to survival. However, previous studies (not as rigorous as this one) had found lower expenditures on care and also confirmed the higher mortality in for-profit units.

### Nursing Homes

About two-thirds of U.S. nursing homes are investor-owned, mostly by large chains, and about one-fourth are owned by private non-profit organizations; the remainder (about 7 percent) are owned by government agencies. Most nursing home income is derived from Medicaid and from out-of-pocket private payments, and these payments are based on standard per diem charges. Although payments may vary according to the level of nursing needed by patients, and in the case of self-paying patients, according to the amenities provided, most nursing home income is relatively fixed per patient. Facilities therefore generate net income according to the "efficiency" with which they administer care. All else being equal, the less they spend on staffing and other services, the more profit they are likely to make. The financial incentives essentially resemble those for dialysis units.

What, then, is the difference between for-profit and not-for-profit facilities in terms of quality of care? A published study of all certified U.S. nursing homes, based on government data collected in 1998, gives a clear answer: Quality deficiencies in patient care identified by state inspection were 56 percent more common in private for-profit than in private not-for-profit facilities and 43 percent more prevalent than in public facilities.[21] When only deficiencies considered by inspectors to be serious were tallied, for-profits had 40 percent more citations than non-profits, and 36 percent more than public nursing homes. Nurse staffing at investor-owned facilities (hours of nursing service per patient bed) was 32 percent lower in investor-owned homes than in non-profit homes, and 23 percent lower than in public facilities. Other, less definitive studies have in general confirmed these conclusions and have also found higher rates of medical complications and death in for-profit facilities.

These findings are in general accord with those described in the kidney dialysis study. When prices are fixed by payers, as they are in nursing homes and dialysis centers, for-profit health care facilities make their profits by reducing expenditures on services, that is, by attempting to be more "efficient" than their competitors. This, unfortunately, risks lowering the quality of care, which may not become apparent until careful comparative studies are done.

### Summary of the Empirical Data

When medical services are not pre-specified and payment is not fixed (as in most ambulatory services and many types of hospital care), investor-owned facilities tend to provide more expensive services to those who are insured and can pay the charges. This raises health expenditures. The quality of care in such facilities is no better than in not-for-profit facilities, and may sometimes be worse. Furthermore, as judged by their higher administrative and overhead expenses, investor-owned facilities are less efficient than not-for-profit or public institutions, meaning that they spend more to produce outcomes that are no better. On the other hand, when medical services and payment are predetermined (as with kidney dialysis and nursing home care), investor-owned facilities spend less on services than not-for-profit providers, and in so doing they lower the quality of care.

Thus, the best available empirical data are consistent with the conclusion that in health care, the business imperative to make profits does not produce the social benefits claimed by market advocates. Instead, it increases costs; it may also jeopardize quality or aggravate the system's inequity. Sometimes it even manages to do all three. When private insurers, health care facilities, and physicians treat health care as a commercial enterprise, the result is what the United States has now—an excessively expensive, inefficient system of uneven quality, which is less accessible to the poor and uninsured.

The effects of commercialization of our health care system have not been limited to the investor-owned sector. The presence of investors and investor-owned businesses has changed the culture of the entire system and affected the behavior of the private not-for-profit sector as well. Therefore, differences between the two should be seen merely as differences in the degree to which investor-owned and not-for-profit institutions respond to the same economic forces. If commercialization has driven up medical costs, reduced access for the uninsured, and jeopardized quality, as I have argued, most private not-for-profit institutions must also share in the responsibility, although the investor-owned institutions have led the way.

## Insurance Plans

To this point, the empirical comparisons between investor-owned and not-for-profit organizations have concerned institutions that deliver care, such as hospitals, dialysis centers, and nursing homes. Nothing has been said about the very important part of the health care system that is "upstream" from the delivery of care, that is, the insurance plans. They pay the providers for care, often (in "managed care" plans) trying to regulate the care itself by deciding what they will pay for and discouraging primary care physicians from the use of hospitals and expensive technology. Are there comparisons between investor-owned and private not-for-profit insurance plans that could shed further light on how investor ownership affects the cost, efficiency, or quality of the health care system? 

Unfortunately, data on this are scarce. Wide variations among groups covered, benefits offered, and payments required of beneficiaries make comparisons of premiums, health care outcomes, and consumer satisfaction in investor-owned and not-for-profit plans almost impossible to interpret. The problem is further complicated by frequent changes in plans and beneficiaries. Employers often change the insurance plans offered to their employees as they constantly shop for better deals. In my opinion, there is only one comparative measure that is meaningful here—the percent of the premium that is retained by the insurance plan for its administrative expenses and profits before it pays providers for the care they give to beneficiaries. By this measure there is a clear difference between investor-owned and not-for-profit plans. As revealed in their annual reports and widely confirmed by all research on this subject, investor-owned plans take roughly 10 to 25 percent of the premium before paying providers, whereas not-for-profit plans take only 5 to 10 percent. This means, of course, that a higher fraction of the premium of not-for-profit plans goes to providers, and it suggests that beneficiaries of non-profit plans get more health care for the same total health expenditure. Incidentally, Medicare, the largest public insurance plan, reports spending less than 3 percent of its total expenditures on administration.

Investor-owned insurance plans add substantial overhead costs to the health care system, without producing commensurate benefits. Ten percent of total expenditures on for-profit private insurance (which is the average difference between the overhead of for-profit and private not-for-profit plans) would probably represent at least

$50 or $60 billion, an expense that cannot be justified by any unique value the for-profit plans add to the health care system. And this very conservative figure does not even consider the additional huge savings that would follow from consolidation of all insurance functions into a single, non-profit system and the elimination of medical billing.

## Billing Fraud

Billing fraud contributes to the cost of health care in both the public and private sectors, but its total extent can only be guessed. There are many kinds of fraud, and the guilty parties include physicians and other health personnel, as well as business corporations and hospitals. Some say that as much as 5 to 10 percent of all insurance payments are generated by fraudulent or other kinds of improper claims. The U.S. Attorney's offices have been focusing particular attention on suspicious Medicare and Medicaid claims by hospitals and have indicted and fined far more for-profit than not-for-profit hospitals for misconduct.[22] In a few highly publicized cases, large investor-owned hospital chains have been indicted and forced to settle for huge sums, sometimes hundreds of millions of dollars or more, and this has resulted in major shake-ups in corporate organization and executive management.

Although there have been far fewer such revelations in the not-for-profit sector, the available data do not allow any firm conclusions about the relative culpability of for-profit and not-for-profit hospital management because investigations into billing practices have not been randomly initiated. What is clear, however, is that the opportunities and the incentives to maximize income in a commercialized and competitive marketplace have tempted some hospitals in both the for-profit and not-for-profit sectors to bill insurers for as much as possible, even when they may be crossing the bounds of the law. When competition for big money is involved, some chicanery seems sure to follow. Fraud is, therefore, one of the inevitable consequences of a commercialized health care system. A reformed system in which billing procedures and incentives to maximize profits were largely eliminated would undoubtedly reduce losses due to fraud.

## The Role of Physicians in the "Cost Explosion"

So far in this chapter, I have been talking about medical care institutions as if they independently determine the behavior of the health care system. They do not. Physicians make most of the decisions to use the resources of medical institutions. Although they receive barely more than one-fifth of all the money spent on personal medical care, physicians control most of what happens in health care through their recommendations, orders, prescriptions, and interventions.

It is true that physicians on a hospital staff do not determine charges or, often, not even the services the hospital will provide. However, they have a great influence on hospital policies because they control hospital admissions and medical care, and they advise hospital management on the acquisition of new technology and equipment. If a hospital's services are unnecessarily expensive, its medical staff is either benefiting from that or for other reasons has chosen to ignore the problem.

But it is not simply doctors' behavior in hospitals and other health facilities that has contributed to the high costs of medical care. Many physicians in their office practice have become more focused on defending and enhancing their income than ever before, and their entrepreneurial behavior contributes to the growing influence of business incentives on medical costs. I have already discussed how doctors have become part of the "medical-industrial complex" in Chapter 1 and described in detail one startling example of this phenomenon in the office treatment of back pain. Such examples abound and are the subject of a growing literature.[23] Although vulnerable to the incentives and economic demands of the marketplace in which they must practice, physicians still have wide latitude in how they use the vast resources of the health care system. They must acknowledge their contribution to rising health expenditures, and they have a major responsibility in helping to solve the problem.

Studies of what is called "small area variations" in Medicare expenditures provide quantitative empirical evidence in support of this contention. For many years, John Wennberg and his colleagues at the Dartmouth Medical Center[24] have been meticulously analyzing records of Medicare payments across the country to compare expenditures on certain medical and surgical procedures across small geographic regions. Their massive database reveals per capita variations of as much as 250 percent in these expenditures, which cannot be explained by any demographic or medical reasons, and which are not reflected in different medical outcomes. These variations seem to be correlated best with the availability of medical and surgical specialists in the areas and apparently reflect local differences in the way medicine is practiced rather than variations in medical need. In short, these data convincingly demonstrate what most physicians know from their own experience: that doctors have a powerful influence on the medical services provided.

When they are paid on a fee-for-service basis and when there are strong economic incentives to maximize their income, the presence of specialists will certainly increase expenditures. In effect, through their choice of tests and procedures, doctors create what economists would term a "demand" for their own services. That is why I contend that physicians play an important part in generating medical expenditures, and why they must take the lead in devising a solution to the problem.

# 3

## THE REVOLT OF THE PAYERS

> Last year, General Motors spent $5.3 billion on health
> care. By 2008, it will likely spend more on health care
> in the U.S. than on its hourly-worker payroll.
>
> —DETROIT NEWS, SEPTEMBER 26, 2006

> This is a national issue and needs to be addressed in
> that light. . . . We can't bet the company on somebody
> stepping up to address this in Washington. We're go-
> ing after it ourselves.
>
> —RICK WAGONER, CEO,
> GENERAL MOTORS, SEPTEMBER 2006

THE RISING HEALTH CARE EXPENDITURES THAT BEGAN IN THE
late 1960s quickly became a problem for the third-party payers,
that is, the government and business employers. In 1970, the
Nixon administration called the situation a "crisis" and began seeking ways to control what threatened to become a runaway inflation
that might destabilize the federal budget. At the same time, businesses started to look for an escape from the constantly rising premiums they were paying for their employees' health insurance.
Thus began what could be called "the revolt of the payers." Rather
than simply accept the bills from doctors and hospitals, both public
and private payers tried to impose their own financial arrangements

on the system in an attempt to curb expenditures. This "revolt" has continued to the present, with payers trying a variety of methods to contain their costs. Except for transient leveling-off periods in the mid-1980s and the late 1990s, the tide of health care costs in both the public and private sectors has shown no signs of significant slowing in response to these efforts (Figure 1).

## HMOs and the Revolt of the Payers in the Private Sector

Employers rebelled against the unpredictable and uncontrolled increases in premiums for the indemnity-type of insurance they were buying for their employees. This had required them to pay whatever the insurance plans demanded for their costs, plus profits. Insurers within the indemnity model had little incentive to hold costs down. Employers wanted a different kind of insurance, with more predictable costs and a better accounting of benefits received. In response, a new and largely investor-owned insurance industry arose, which contracted with employers to provide "managed care" insurance plans. "Managed care" insurance is a general term used to describe plans that exercise some control over the quantity and quality of the services received by beneficiaries, rather than simply paying the bills submitted by providers. By accepting responsibility for controlling costs and assuming the financial risk if they failed, the plans were able to guarantee a certain range of medical benefits at a prepaid price, which was precisely what employers were looking for.

The first type of prepaid managed care to gain wide currency in the private insurance market was the so-called HMO (or health maintenance organization), a name and concept introduced to the Nixon administration by Dr. Paul Ellwood.[1] Employers either selected an HMO plan for their workers or gave employees a choice among a few. Employers paid about 80 percent of the premiums, and employees the rest. Benefits varied, but they usually included payment of doctor and hospital bills for employees and their families, and sometimes for retirees. They also usually included certain preventive services that were supposed to promote "health maintenance." In addition to a share of the premium, beneficiaries were often required to pay "co-payments" for services as they received them. HMOs controlled medical expenditures by requiring beneficiaries to select a primary care physician from among a panel of local doctors under contract with the plan. Primary care doctors had to approve all referrals to specialists and had to get approval from the plan before admitting patients to the hospital or prescribing expensive tests and medications. Primary care physicians were usually paid on a per capita basis and could refer only to the selected specialists on the plan's panel, who had agreed to accept discounted fees.

Most physicians had to deal with many different plans, which compounded the administrative work for them and their office staff. The specialists and the hospitals to which beneficiaries could be referred also had greater administrative expenses in dealing with multiple plans. Expenditures, specialist referral patterns, and the use of hospitals by the primary care physicians were monitored by each plan, which usually rewarded the primary care doctors for frugal practice behavior and penalized them financially for the opposite.

There were many variations in HMO organization and procedures, but I have described here the typical arrangement, in which physicians practiced independently in their own offices and usually signed contracts with several different HMO insurance plans to care for the plans' beneficiaries. "Staff-model" HMOs employed their own primary care physicians. "Group-model" plans contracted with multi-specialty physician groups that provided all primary care, and most specialized care as well. A few of the biggest group-model plans, such as Kaiser-Permanente, owned their own hospitals.

In America, the idea of prepaid insurance for medical care dates back to eighteenth-century Boston, but its first modern appearance was in 1929, when the Ross-Loos Clinic, a salaried multi-specialty group practice, contracted with the City of Los Angeles to provide care for unionized employees in the Department of Water and Power. However, it wasn't until later that the concept took hold, when Dr. Sidney Garfield and Mr. Edgar Kaiser devised a plan to provide comprehensive medical care for the Kaiser Corporation's workers at the Grand Coulee Dam and in the World War II Kaiser shipyards. The Garfield-Kaiser plan subsequently developed into the giant Kaiser-Permanente Health system in California. This concept combined a non-profit prepaid insurance system (Kaiser Health Plan) with a salaried multi-specialty group of physicians (Permanente Medical Group) and several Kaiser-owned hospitals.[2] It provided a new style of integrated medical care combined with medical insurance, which was soon copied by a number of other large health organizations such as the Group Health Cooperative of Puget Sound and the Health Insurance Plan of New York.

What Paul Ellwood had in mind in the 1970s was a national network of many similar, but much smaller, prepaid health insurance plans, which would compete for contracts with employers and would compete for beneficiaries that were covered by Medicare and Medicaid. They would have a variety of different kinds of ownership and a variety of contractual arrangements with physicians and hospitals, but they would all be competing on the basis of fully disclosed prices and reports of medical outcomes. The HMO Act of 1973 encouraged the formation and growth of private HMOs through federal grants, contracts, and loans. This was government's first attempt to control health expenditures, and it was directed primarily at relieving the problems facing employers in the private sector. The legislation was strongly supported by business and provided major impetus for the adoption of HMO plans by many employers.

The essence of the HMO idea was to control expenditures and enable employers to pay up front for an agreed-upon package of medical services for their employees. But to be profitable, HMOs had to limit the freedom of beneficiaries to consult physicians of their choice. They also had to use financial incentives and penalties to get physicians to practice in what management considered a cost-effective style. They bargained aggressively with physicians and hospitals to lower their fees, and they employed teams of nurses as "case managers," to promote early discharge from the hospital. In short, HMOs could fairly be said to favor the financial interests of employers and the insurance company over those of patients and doctors. It was an arrangement that would inevitably cause a backlash.

The administrators of the new HMO plans claimed they improved the quality of care by eliminating the risks and expense of unnecessary procedures and prolonged hospitalizations, by monitoring physician performance, by "case management," and by paying for certain preventive measures. However, these policies were perceived by most physicians and patients as restrictions on care, really designed for the financial benefit of the insurers and employers. After all, the great majority of the new HMO plans were investor owned. They were businesses, whose substantial profits depended in part on avoiding coverage of workers with chronic illnesses likely to be costly. They also made money by minimizing the use of hospitals and expensive services. Physicians were expected to obtain advance approval for elective hospital admissions and expensive diagnostic or therapeutic procedures, and such requests were sometimes refused or allowed only after appeals and delays, dissuading many doctors from even trying. Critics said that the for-profit HMOs had a financial conflict of interest with their members—and they were right.

Not surprisingly, these new investor-owned HMOs had higher corporate administrative costs than the older indemnity insurance plans. However, they used fewer of their premium dollars for payment of medical services and could therefore keep their premiums competitively low, while boasting to their stockholders that their "medical losses" (that is, their payments to providers for care of their beneficiaries) were also low. Despite their claims to be improving the health care of their beneficiaries, there were no convincing data to prove the case. The relatively rapid turnover of beneficiaries undermined the rationale for preventive care and cast serious doubt on whether patients or the plan would get any long-term benefits from such care. Nevertheless, the HMO idea initially had broad appeal to employers, who chose the insurance plans for their workers or offered them a choice from among a selected few.[3] It was also incorporated into the plan for health care reform that was intended to be the centerpiece of domestic policy in the Clinton administration that came to power in 1992.

## The Clinton Plan for Health Reform

The ill-fated national plan proposed by the Clinton administration in 1993 was based on the concept of "managed competition" among HMOs, as first developed by Alain C. Enthoven, a Stanford Business School economist.[4] Although Enthoven advocated allowing market forces to control prices and total costs, the Clinton team believed that the market would need considerable government regulation to ensure nearly universal coverage and control costs. They therefore included in the plan a global budget cap and many other regulatory provisions that Enthoven and many conservatives thought would interfere with the free play of the market. Nevertheless, some of the largest employers, eager to control their health care costs, at first supported the proposal.

But the hostility of the private insurance and pharmaceutical industries, coupled with the general fear of government regulation shared by almost all business managers, turned the business community and their friends in Congress against the plan. Some professional medical organizations (for example, the American Academy of Pediatrics, the American College of Physicians, the American Academy of Obstetricians and Gynecologists, and the American Academy of Family Physicians) were initially attracted to the proposal, but the administration's relations with rank-and-file practicing physicians was never very good, and at the end, the AMA and most practitioners joined U.S. business in opposing what was increasingly caricatured as "big government" dictating private choices in health care. The arcane details of the proposed bill and its excessive length made it almost impossible for most people to understand, thus further complicating the Clinton administration's task in selling it to the public. So it was hardly a surprise when, in September 1994, the proposal died in Congress without ever coming to a floor vote.[5]

Even before the official pronouncement of the Clinton plan's demise, pressures from employers for better control of costs had created a booming new competitive market for independent private insurance plans based on the HMO concept. The late 1980s and early 1990s saw a great increase in the popularity of investor-owned managed care plans among employers. Many new insurance businesses were started, many older indemnity-type mutual and not-for-profit insurance companies were converted to for-profit managed care plans, and many acquisitions and mergers created large new entities: for-profit health insurance firms. It was a transformation of the private health insurance market that in many ways resembled the change that had occurred some fifteen or twenty years earlier among private hospitals, when investor-owned hospital chains first appeared on the scene.

For a few years during the early 1990s, when HMO-type insurance was spreading, the rise in private health expenditures was controlled (Figure 1). Employers were gratified to see their premiums hold steady, and even decrease slightly, as insurance payments to doctors and hospitals slowed. However, this phase proved to be only temporary.

## The Decline of HMOs and the Rise of PPOs

By the beginning of the new century, the continued rise in billing by providers forced insurers once again to increase their premiums, and expenditures on health care resumed their steady climb (Figure 1). Curtailment of hospital admissions, controls on expensive diagnostic procedures, and discounting of payments to physicians and hospitals could be taken only so far by the private insurance plans before being overridden by the ever-expanding costs of the U.S. health care system. HMOs simply could not stem the tide, and this reduced their appeal to employers.

But even if HMOs had been more successful in containing costs, they would still have faced unyielding opposition from other quarters. Resistance from patients and physicians, who did not like the limitations on medical practice imposed by HMOs, was forcing employers to abandon these plans. Physicians were outspoken in their criticism of the red tape involved in conforming to the multiple requirements of the different plans, while patients brought lawsuits against the plans for denying payment for services considered medically necessary by their physicians. Increasing demand by employees for more freedom to choose their own physicians, and increasing demand by physicians for more freedom of clinical decisionmaking, forced employers to look beyond HMOs and ask health insurers for a less painful kind of managed care. A major reason for the effectiveness of the employee backlash against managed care was the tight labor market during the economic boom of the late 1990s. Employers had to be responsive to their workers' concerns if they wanted to find new employees.

The private health insurance industry was not about to give up its lucrative business with employers, so as the use of the unpopular HMO-type of managed care declined, it promoted another, much less restrictive form of managed care, which it had been offering for some time. These more liberal plans were known as "preferred provider organization" (PPO) insurance. In such plans, members selected a primary care provider from among a panel of physicians that was approved by the insurance plan, but they were free to consult specialists and did not need advance approval from their primary care physician. However, they could only choose specialists from among a selected list of "preferred providers" who had agreed to accept the insurer's fees or other payments. With the spread of PPOs and decline of HMOs, there were fewer complaints from employees about denials or delays in services or restrictions on the choice of physicians. But costs began to rise very rapidly again because beneficiaries now had unimpeded access to the expensive services of specialists.

Employers are presently being forced to use other means of controlling their health care expenditures. They are taking a direct, if more brutal, approach: They are abandoning their earlier commitment to pay most of the cost of health care by unilaterally curtailing contributions to their employees' health benefits and shifting a larger share of the expense to workers, or they are capping their contribution and allowing employees to bear the full brunt of rising premiums. A growing number of employees are shifting to low-premium, high-deductible insurance, coupled with health savings accounts. Some employers are cutting their previous support of retirees' benefits, while others are turning to new hiring arrangements that do not include any health benefits. Except in a few areas, the labor supply has expanded considerably since the 1990s, and employers don't have to be as concerned about maintaining fringe benefits in order to find employees.

Workers, fearful of losing their jobs in a market now much less favorable to those seeking work, cannot fight back, and their unions can do little to reverse the trend. When rising health costs force big corporations to reduce benefits and lay off workers in order to help the company survive in an unfavorable market, the union has little choice but to acquiesce. In short, employers are "solving" the problem of their health insurance costs by simply walking away from it, dumping the problem into the laps of their workers. Employers may argue that workers, as the direct recipients of care, should be more effective at reining in costs than management (part of the theory of "consumer-driven health care"), but the ugly fact remains that the ranks of the uninsured and the underinsured are swelling, as responsibility for coverage is gradually being shifted from employers to their employees.

General Motors is a striking example of the desperate need of large employers to control their health care costs. In 2005, GM spent $5.3 billion on the health care costs of its 1.1 million workers and retirees and their families, or over $5,000 per year for each GM-insured person.[6] That adds an estimated $1,525 to the average price of every vehicle the company builds in the United States. By comparison, GM spends only $1,385 per year for each insured person in its Canadian plant, which adds only $197 to the average cost of each vehicle assembled there. The difference is due primarily to Canada's national health system, which pays most of the medical bills of Canadian workers. Toyota, GM's largest competitor, spends only $97 on workers' health care for each vehicle it builds in Japan.

Health costs make it almost impossible for GM to be price competitive with Toyota or other foreign manufacturers. The company is now engaged in a struggle to survive against its competition. "Because of its aging work force and army of retirees, GM has reached a health care crisis before the rest of the country," the *Detroit News* reported on September 26, 2006. It quoted Warren Buffett as saying that "GM is a health and benefits company with an auto company attached." As health expenditures for other large businesses continue to rise, that description may become more generally applicable.

Like many other big companies, GM acts as its own insurer, taking the risk of paying for each of its workers' health bills. It tries to control its costs by negotiating prices with doctors and hospitals, arranging convenient and inexpensive company-run ambulatory services and walk-in clinics to avoid unnecessary hospitalizations and emergency room visits, using "case-managers," and encouraging its workers to adopt healthier lifestyles. Now, like other U.S. auto manufacturers faced with declining sales and rising health costs, GM is cutting the size of its workforce and the benefits it provides them, in a struggle to avoid bankruptcy. Other U.S. industries are undoubtedly wondering whether their rising health costs will soon put them in a similar position.

## The Revolt of the Payers in the Public Sector

Although government was quick to recognize a health cost "crisis" just a few years after implementation of its Medicare and Medicaid programs, its initial response was confined to legislation in 1973 that helped HMO-type insurance plans become established in the private sector.[7] There was little or no immediate effect on government insurance programs, which continued to pay hospitals and physicians on the traditional fee-for-service indemnification basis. But as government expenditures on health programs mounted, the need for control became more urgent. Payments to hospitals were the largest part of the federal burden, so they were the first target. Medicare Part A, which had initially paid hospitals' itemized per diem charges, changed to a new payment system. Legislation passed in 1982 and 1983 required that payments be determined according to the diagnosis of each patients' medical problem, not by the number of days in the hospital or the cost of the various services provided. For each diagnosis, there would be a specified payment to cover the entire admission, regardless of its length or the individual services provided. The legislation also set limits on the rate of increase in payments, and adjusted payments to local wage costs and to each hospital's costs for education and community services. This so-called "DRG" (diagnosis-related groups) system applied only to inpatient services at general hospitals, not to ambulatory (outpatient) services or to children's, psychiatric, or rehabilitation hospitals.

Nevertheless, this reform had a major impact on hospital bills, and public expenditures on health services slowed in the mid-1980s.

The DRG payment system was also adopted by many private insurers, resulting in a slowing of the rise in private expenditures on hospitalization. As a result, total health spending almost leveled off for a few years in the 1980s (Figure 1). The effects of the DRG system on hospital behavior were predictable. The average length of stay in general hospitals plummeted, more diagnostic studies were carried out on an ambulatory basis, and patients were discharged much earlier, to continue their convalescence at home or in long-term facilities. Patients were discharged "quicker and sicker," often to their discomfort and the chagrin of their physicians. Hospitals began to employ nurse "case managers" to monitor recovering patients and remind their physicians to get them out of the hospital as soon as possible.

In teaching hospitals, where medical students and young residents had traditionally learned their clinical skills by examining and observing hospitalized patients during all phases of their illness and by assisting in their diagnosis and treatment, the rapidity with which patients were now hustled in and out of the hospital compromised the educational experience.[8] Major teaching hospitals, formerly centers of education as well as care, were filled with a higher than ever percentage of patients who were acutely ill or undergoing major surgical procedures. Hospitals had to be more concerned with controlling costs, and they were less able to cross-subsidize the expenses of providing medical education. As a result, students had less chance to observe, senior staff physicians less time to teach, and medical residents were so busy writing admission notes, scheduling procedures on their patients, and tending to their acute medical problems that they had little time for education. This problem remains unresolved to this day, although many medical schools and teaching hospitals are actively experimenting with new solutions.

Not surprisingly, some hospitals tried to game the DRG reimbursement system through what is known as "diagnostic creep." They systematically inflated their income from DRGs by "upgrading" diagnostic categories—changing low-paying diagnoses to closely related diagnoses that are reimbursed at higher rates. However, DRGs forced hospitals to use their resources more economically, and that resulted in the trimming of unused bed capacity and the closing of some unneeded hospitals. To defend their income, hospitals shifted more services to their ambulatory departments, where DRGs did not apply. The number of ambulatory surgery centers, which were not subject to the DRG system, increased greatly during the 1980s and 1990s. Now, almost half of all the surgery that was formerly performed in hospitals is done on an ambulatory basis in ambulatory surgery centers and in doctors' offices. In the same manner, much of the expensive diagnostic imaging (for example, CT scans and MRIs) is now done in doctors' offices, in freestanding "imaging centers," or in ambulatory divisions affiliated with hospitals. Home health care and nursing home care have also increased.

Government has also tried to rein in its payments to physicians under Part B of Medicare. Legislation that took effect in 1992 established the so-called "RBRVS" (resource-based relative-value scale) system to replace the older arrangement for paying doctors. Under the new system, each physician service is assigned a "relative value" based on the time, skill, and intensity of effort it requires. Then a conversion factor, corrected for local prices, is applied to these values, to calculate the fee that Medicare will pay. The relative values were supposed to improve what was widely perceived as an imbalance between excessive compensation for technical procedures and underpayment for more personal, "cognitive" services requiring more time with patients. The conversion factor was intended to control the total payment to physicians, which had been increasing as rapidly as the payment to facilities. Like the DRG system for hospital payment, the government's RBRVS physician payment system was also adopted by many private insurers, and it influenced the fees paid to physicians by private insurers. Together with the managed care efforts of HMOs, this new physician payment method probably contributed to the stabilization of total health expenditures for several years in the mid-1990s (Figure 1).

The net effect of the new physician payment system on the availability of primary care and specialty physicians' services is complicated. The many factors causing the proportion of specialists to grow, the rising expense of new technology, and the increasing overhead costs of practice make it difficult to draw conclusions. Suffice it to say that the relative value scale has not had any dramatic effect on the continuing large gap between the income of specialists and that of primary care physicians or on the continuing replacement of primary care physicians by specialists. And neither has the use of the conversion factor been very effective in controlling total expenditures on physician services, which for the past two decades have been slowly rising as a percentage of total health expenditures. However, the AMA claims that the average income of physicians, corrected for inflation, has not increased, and that the increase in physician numbers largely accounts for the rising total expenditures on physicians' services. Proposals by Congress to ratchet down physicians' fees in Medicare are invariably met by resistance from the AMA, which argues that failure to at least keep up with the ever-increasing overhead expenses of medical office practice will force many physicians to refuse caring for new Medicare patients.

This account of the government's attempt to control its health care expenditures would not be complete without some mention of its misbegotten efforts to enroll Medicare beneficiaries in private managed care plans. Beginning with the Nixon administration in the early 1970s, and continuing to the present, Republican-promoted policies have been aimed at helping private insurers persuade those over sixty-five to exchange their traditional fee-for-service Medicare coverage for approved managed care plans that would be paid by Medicare.

At first, Medicare paid participating plans a premium that was equal to 95 percent of the average per capita Medicare expenditure in each geographic area, and for this the plans were required to cover all the standard Medicare benefits plus whatever additional benefits might be required to attract the customers. The attraction for beneficiaries included such additional benefits as free checkups and some outpatient drugs. Also, the plans required beneficiaries to pay less in out-of-pocket co-payments and deductibles, which are part of traditional Medicare and often cause recipients to buy supplemental insurance. The attraction of this deal for the private plans was supposed to be access to new markets and the opportunity to show that they could provide more benefits to the elderly than the fee-for-service traditional government-run Medicare system. It was expected they would be able to make a profit even when paid at a rate 5 percent below the average per capita Medicare expenditures in their geographic area. It was, after all, part of conservative dogma that private enterprise would be more efficient than government in managing health care. Outsourcing health insurance to the private sector would not only save the government a little money; it would also provide the elderly with more benefits.

But the plan did not live up to those expectations. What happened was an instructive lesson in how private investor-owned insurance companies conduct their business and how corporate interests influence government policy. In the absence of any effective regulations to prevent "cherry-picking" by the private plans, they recruited into the new arrangements (called "Medicare plus Choice" or Medicare "Plan C") Medicare beneficiaries who were disproportionately younger and healthier than those who remained in the traditional

Medicare system. Despite this advantage, many private plans that were unable to make their expected profits abruptly terminated their contracts. Government tried to keep the private insurers interested by increasing the premium rate to levels *higher* than the average Medicare per capita expenditures in a given area. However, many beneficiaries were dissatisfied with the plans and began to disenroll in large numbers. The number of "Medicare plus Choice" beneficiaries, which at first had increased rapidly, reached a peak of about 6 million—or 16 percent of the Medicare population—in the year 2000, but since then has declined.

The Medicare Modernization Act was passed by the narrowest of margins at the end of 2003 after intense pressure from the White House and from drug and insurance industry lobbyists. It included funds for private managed care plans, now called "Medicare Advantage." To encourage Medicare beneficiaries to switch their coverage, the private plans offered prescription drug coverage and preventive medicine services not included in traditional Medicare, as well as much more choice of physicians and hospitals than had been available under HMO-type coverage. Enrollment in these plans has increased, but the percentage of total Medicare beneficiaries making the change still remains low, at about 12 percent. Moreover, these plans have continued to be more expensive per capita than traditional Medicare. Contrary to the prediction of private sector enthusiasts, in 2005 the private insurers charged the federal government on average 11 to 12 percent more per beneficiary than the government spent on Medicare beneficiaries in the same geographic region. However, there are no good data comparing the relative age and health status of those with private and public coverage, so the full significance of this disparity cannot be assessed.

The main objective of the Medicare Modernization Act of 2003 was to provide an elective prescription drug benefit ("Medicare Part D") for patients who chose to remain on Medicare but wanted coverage for prescription drugs. Because its legislative sponsors apparently were persuaded of the greater wisdom and efficiency of private markets, and because the pharmaceutical industry lobbied very hard for this provision, the bill outsourced the administration of the drug program to private insurance companies and specifically empowered them, rather than Medicare, to negotiate prices with the manufacturers.[9] The legislation ensured large profits for drug manufacturers, denying Medicare any role in bargaining for prices, despite the fact that the Veterans Administration (VA) and the armed services have that authority in negotiating for the purchase of the drugs they use. Official estimates place the total costs to Medicare over the next ten years at over $500 billion, hence the sharp upward inflection in projected Medicare spending at the year 2006 in Figure 1.

Critics have suggested that much taxpayer money could be saved if the program were entirely administered by Medicare and if that agency, rather than private insurance plans, were allowed to negotiate drug prices. Drugs presently constitute only about 12 percent of health costs, but expenditures are rising more rapidly than most other parts of the health care economy.[10] Rising expenditures on prescription drugs are a part of the general problem of health care costs, and the controversy over the bill is a good example of the differences among policymakers on whether the private market or government regulation is the best way to control costs.

I have not described government's attempts to control rising costs in the Medicaid program because the story would have to be more complicated, technical, and detailed than would be appropriate for this book. Unlike Medicare, Medicaid covers a large and constantly changing number of different categories of beneficiaries, and its expenditures are affected by differing state policies. In addition to the general methods used by Medicare, state Medicaid programs have tried to limit their costs by changes in benefits and eligibility, even while struggling to respond to federal mandates to expand coverage of the growing number of uninsured poor children and their parents. But the bottom line has been essentially the same as for Medicare—constantly increasing total expenditures at a rate that is straining most state budgets as well as the federal Centers for Medicare and Medicaid Services.

## Why Have the Cost-Control Strategies Failed?

Although the annual percentage increase in health care expenditures has been lower in the past few years than previously, it remains intolerably high in both the public and the private sectors. Some of the recent decline in the rate of inflation in expenditures could be attributed to the cost-control strategies I have described, but the problem has by no means been solved, particularly when viewed in the context of the increasing numbers of uninsured and underinsured people. Health expenditures continue to grow more rapidly than the rest of the economy and to threaten the economic viability of government and business.

So then, how to explain the inability of both private and public payers to keep the growth of health expenditures within acceptable limits? The answer is obvious. In a commercialized health care system in which physicians and clinical facilities are still largely reimbursed on a fee-for-service basis, there is a powerful incentive to provide more services and to favor more expensive services over simpler ones so long as the patient or an insurance plan can pay. Even when fees are discounted or bundled (as with the "DRG" payment method), the number and choice of services remains largely under the control of the provider, not the payer, and the providers' economic interests drive up the bills. Although managed care, particularly the HMO version, is potentially an effective method of controlling inflation, neither patients nor physicians were able to tolerate the restrictions on clinical practice imposed by

HMOs, and this strategy had to be abandoned in favor of a more relaxed (and expensive version) of managed care—that is, PPOs.

When a large enough part of the system becomes an investor-owned industry, continuous growth of revenue (meaning increased expenditure on health care) is a fundamental imperative for the providers. Furthermore, insurance coverage reduces the concerns of beneficiaries about expenditures. And given the fact that the demand for most medical services is determined by professional medical judgment, neither consumers nor payers have much leverage in controlling expenditures. That is especially true if the medical judgment is exercised by physicians who benefit financially from each service that is provided. It stands to reason that a commercially motivated health care system will be constantly pushing for the delivery of more services, because the providers who profit from increased expenditures will resist all efforts at cost control. So long as that system remains, we cannot expect much from attempts at controlling expenditures.

## Some Untested Proposals for Cost Control

*Rationing.* Some economists, seeing the contribution to rising expenditures made by the increased use of expensive new technology, believe that the deliberate and systematic rationing of this technology is the only solution to the control of costs.[11] They say we should develop a method of evaluating new technology and use it to prevent reimbursement by public or private insurance for procedures and equipment that are of little value. Advocates further argue that to have any significant effect on expenditures, rationing would have to include much technology that might be helpful to some degree, but not enough to warrant the expense. And, to be ethically acceptable, rationing would have to be explicit, public, and uniformly applied. It could not be like the implicit, unacknowledged, and often almost random kind of rationing now so common in this country, which is determined by racial and cultural factors and by ability to pay.

In my opinion, developing an explicit system of rationing like that would be close to impossible. Even its strongest advocates admit that there is now no effective and acceptable way to make and implement rationing decisions, nor are there any solutions on the horizon. The multitude of individual clinical considerations with which physicians would have to struggle, the probable reluctance of government officials to defend their rationing policies publicly, and the inevitable pressures from vested interests and influential patients to circumvent the regulations almost guarantee that rationing would never be widely accepted in the United States. Furthermore, in the absence of an effective method for regulating the development of all new technology, I cannot see how rationing the use of individual technologies would control expenditures. Decisions on individual technologies would be under constant challenge as supporting evidence changed, new technologies entered the market, and existing technologies were refined. So the notion of an orderly and scientific rationing process, explicitly identified as such, and managed by experts who would be free of political and commercial influence and could persuade doctors and patients to accept their judgments, is unrealistic.

I very much doubt that explicit, compulsory rationing on a scale large enough to significantly limit health care spending will ever be put to a national test. That is not to say that we don't need a better system for the clinical evaluation of technology. We certainly do, but assuming each new technology has been approved by a competent public evaluation of its safety and effectiveness before entering the market, judgments about its use in individual cases should be left to doctors and patients. However, we need to be sure that physicians have no incentives to over- or underuse the technology, and no conflicts of interest that might influence their judgment. This will require reforming the health care delivery system. We will also need to set some limits on total expenditures that everyone will have to accept.

*Lowered Expectations.* This proposal has been made in a recent book by Daniel Callahan, a philosopher and one of the founders of the field of bioethics.[12] He agrees with the economists who say that a major cause of health cost inflation is the relentless advance of medical science and technology, and that no cost-containment policy can be successful unless the introduction and use of expensive technology is controlled. To do this, he says, we will have to rethink our notions of limitless and continuous progress in medicine. We must be willing to accept illness and death after a full normal life span of seventy-five to eighty-five years. Instead of using expensive technology in an effort to survive beyond that age, we should concentrate on less costly methods to improve the quality of the years we have been given. Low-technology methods should be used to make the years near the end of life more comfortable, but people should not insist on efforts to extend their lives indefinitely. Callahan advocates less emphasis on developing expensive new technology that only produces marginal benefits and more attention to the relief of symptoms and the treatment of disabilities with less expensive, available methods. He also believes we should devote more resources to preventive medicine and public health.

Much of Callahan's discussion provides a moral argument for a national policy to deal with the probability that there will never be enough resources to pay for all the marginally beneficial but expensive care that some elderly people might want. It is also a call to share what resources we have in order to improve care for all, and a plea for greater realism about the limits of even the most sophisticated care. Since decline and death are unavoidable, Callahan says it is futile to hope that more money spent on searching for new treatments and new technology will protect us from our fate. We should concentrate on helping people live the end of their lives in greater comfort and dignity. Callahan is in favor of avoiding needless expense by improving the efficiency of our health care system and by evaluating the effectiveness of technology. But he does not believe those policies will suffice to control health cost inflation unless they are combined with a widespread lowering of expectations and a willingness to forgo expensive services for the elderly.

I have already said that the proposal to control rising costs through a public policy of explicit rationing based on cost-effectiveness is an illusion—an unworkable idea that would never be accepted. This proposal by Callahan would also never be accepted because it amounts to rationing based on age. In the first place, there is no evidence that elimination of all the "inappropriate" use of expensive technology in the elderly could solve the health cost problem. Although it is true that a substantial portion (about one-third) of all Medicare payments are for treatment in the last six months of life, this hasn't changed significantly over the years. Furthermore, much of that expenditure is undoubtedly made when the outcome of treatment is unknown and the possibility of providing the patient with more years of good quality life is quite real, so it cannot all be considered futile or inappropriate.

There is a real need for more rational and humane treatment of the very old, and the terminally ill, but I doubt that routine limitations of care based exclusively on age, such as Callahan advocates, would be acceptable to the general public, the medical profession, or politicians, and I don't think it is necessary. We Americans believe in medical science and technology. Regardless of our age or illness, and almost regardless of cost, if our physicians think it might help, we will always want the best treatment that modern medicine has to offer. In a different and more efficient health care system, we should be able to afford that.

*Elimination of Expensive Chronic Diseases.* Dr. William B. Schwartz, a distinguished senior academic physician who has been a leading proponent of rationing, wrote an interesting book in 1998,[13] proposing another solution for the constant rise in medical costs. While still advocating rationing as a short-term expedient (admittedly, he says, an imperfect one), he suggests that in the long run, major technical and scientific advances in medicine will eliminate most of the important causes of illness, extend our healthy life span by another forty years, and greatly reduce the need for medical services. He predicts a time, perhaps by the middle of this century, when we will have learned to prevent or cure most expensive diseases.

Schwartz's sanguine prediction about the cost savings to be gained by medical advances is not generally shared; many experts believe that new expenses will simply replace the old. Furthermore, a major epidemic or public health disaster might consume vast resources at any time, thus defeating all efforts at cost control. In any event, U.S. society and most policymakers are primarily concerned about the urgent cost problems we face now. Relief that would not be felt for several more decades is of little comfort to a society that is struggling to cope with today's costs. Even if Schwartz were correct, we cannot wait for his solution. It would not come in time to save a health care system that is on the verge of disaster.

*Malpractice Reform.* The Bush administration and the AMA have identified the costs of the malpractice system as being one of the important causes of the inflation in health care expenditures, and they have urged major reforms. The malpractice system certainly has many problems that need to be fixed, but I can't believe that solving them would have much effect on national health costs. Total direct costs of malpractice litigation include awards to plaintiffs, legal expenses, and insurance company overhead, which are largely covered by the premiums paid to insurers. These are estimated to be approximately $7 billion. Even if these direct costs were totally eliminated, our enormous national health expenditures (now over $2 trillion) would hardly be affected.

But it is argued that there are much larger indirect costs, reflecting expenditures on "defensive" medical practices, that is, procedures done solely, or mainly, for the purpose of avoiding or protecting against litigation in the event of bad outcomes. Indirect costs are unknowable and can only be guessed at. They have been variously estimated to be between $20 and $80 billion. In any case, it is obvious that even the highest estimates of the total cost of the medical liability system are relatively small when compared with the national bill for health care. At the most, the cost of the malpractice system could account for less than 5 percent of total national health expenditures. Furthermore, the elimination of all malpractice-related costs would not do much to change a bill that is relentlessly increasing at a rate that would quickly nullify any savings. In short, while I certainly advocate thoroughgoing reform of our dysfunctional malpractice system, I do not think it warrants serious consideration as a cost-control proposal.

# 4

---

# "CONSUMER-DRIVEN" HEALTH CARE: THE NEW NEW THING

> The right . . . has decided the problem with unafford-
> able health care is that it needs to be *more* unaffordable,
> at least for the people who need it most.
>
> —THE EDITORS OF THE *NEW REPUBLIC*

OF ALL THE PROPOSALS FOR COST CONTROL, THOSE NOW
receiving the most attention are collectively referred to as "consumer-
driven health care" (CDHC). They are the centerpiece of the Bush
administration's program for improving the health care system and
are advocated by conservative think tanks and many economists
and businesspeople. It is too early to evaluate their effect on U.S.
health care, but as of this writing, more than 3 million people have
insurance plans embodying at least some features of CDHC, and
their number is rising.

## Consumer-Driven Health Care: The Three Pillars

As currently used, the term "consumer-driven health care" refers to
various strategies that attempt to create a market for medical care
in which patients, as the "consumers" of medical care, would have

the responsibility for choosing their own services and their own insurance, and would also pay a larger share of the costs. In this new "consumer-driven" market, providers of medical care (physicians, hospitals, clinics, diagnostic facilities, and so on) would compete for patients on the basis of price, quality, and convenience. Like consumers in any service market, patients would have access to all the information they need to make their own health care choices. They would choose, and personally own, their health care insurance. They would select not only their health care insurers and providers but also the particular medical services they want. Since they would be bearing a much larger share of the costs, they would have an incentive to make economical choices and to demand high quality. The desired net result would be a less expensive but higher quality health care system. Advocates for CDHC claim that in our current system, traditional insurance makes beneficiaries indifferent to costs. The best way to curb spending, they say, is to have people pay more of the cost and take more of a role in choosing their own care.

Proponents of the CDHC approach hope to achieve these goals through three reforms. First, patients are required to select and purchase (before taxes) a high-deductible "catastrophic" insurance plan. The plan pays for most of the cost of medical services that exceed the deductible, leaving the cost of everything below the deductible to be paid by patients. The higher the deductible, the lower the premiums for the insurance plan, so people with limited incomes have an incentive to choose plans with high deductibles, despite the greater costs if they become sick. Under current law, plans cannot require total annual out-of-pocket payments for services received (deductibles, plus any additional co-payments) of more than $5,240 for a single beneficiary and $10,500 for families. These limits, which do not include the cost of the insurance premium, should be considered as illustrative only, because they are subject to modification by subsequent legislation.

A second feature of CDHC is a "health savings account" (HSA), which helps to pay the costs of medical services under the insurance plan. This is created by a tax-exempt annual contribution from employers (with optional tax-exempt supplementation by employees), which is wholly owned by the employee and is portable from job to job, as is the insurance policy itself. Current law allows a maximum annual HSA contribution of up to $2,700 for plans covering a single person and up to $5,450 for family plans. These figures will undoubtedly change. The Bush administration has already proposed raising these limits to the level of a plan's maximum deductible. Any part of the HSA not used to pay medical expenses can be invested, tax-exempt, and rolled over annually until age sixty-five. All money from the account that is spent on health care is tax exempt; money used for any other purpose is taxed.

The idea of health savings accounts to be used in conjunction with high-deductible insurance to pay medical costs was popularized in the late 1980s and early 1990s by economist John C. Goodman, president of the conservative National Center for Policy Analysis (NPCA) in Dallas, Texas. The idea was also given impetus by the Cato Institute, a conservative libertarian think tank, which published a book by Goodman and Gerald L. Musgrave in 1992 that expounded the plan in great detail.[1] The plan and the book were endorsed by such conservative stalwarts as Rush Limbaugh, Milton Friedman, William F. Buckley, Jr., and former Senator Phil Gramm (R) of Texas.

The accounts (initially termed "medical savings accounts," or MSAs) were given tax-exempt status in 1996 by federal legislation that was spearheaded by then House Speaker Newt Gingrich. The law limited the numbers of such policies that could be issued and the idea never gained wide acceptance until it was revived under the Bush administration and renamed "health savings account" (HSA). HSAs were created by a provision of the Medicare Modernization Act of 2003, legislation that was primarily designed to extend outpatient prescription drug coverage benefits to Medicare beneficiaries. If employees choose to purchase a high-deductible plan, they receive an annual contribution to their HSA from their employer, which replaces the employer's previous contribution to their health insurance. Employers thus make a defined, and usually smaller, contribution to their employees' standard, managed care health benefits, shifting the rest of the cost to the employee and avoiding the rising premium costs of the low-deductible plans usually offered to their workers. In exchange for the tax-free HSA contribution from their employer, workers assume the cost of the premiums for their high-deductible insurance and take the risk of having to use their HSA to pay the deductible if they or their dependents get sick. Not surprisingly, the CDHC idea has found considerable favor among employers, although the initial response of their employees has been less enthusiastic.

High-deductible medical insurance and tax-exempt HSAs are intended to encourage individuals to choose their own medical care and pay for much of it. CDHC is supposed to provide financial incentives for economical purchasing behavior. But, as Arrow pointed out in 1963,[2] there is such a strong "asymmetry" of information between the providers and consumers of medical care that ordinary market forces cannot be expected to operate. Individuals cannot be prudent shoppers in a medical market because they usually have very little information about the nature of the services they need, or about the comparative prices and quality of available services.

To remedy this situation, advocates of CDHC have proposed a third major reform in the health care system, that is, making all necessary information readily available to consumers of medical care. Through a wide variety of media, including Web sites, guidelines, and articles in magazines and newspapers, government and private sources would convey to the public what they need to know before making health care decisions. Doctors, clinics, hospitals, and other providers would be encouraged—or maybe even required—to disclose their prices and outcomes of treatment, together with any other information that might help potential "customers" make their choices. Advertising to the public about the physicians, facilities, drugs, and procedures available to treat or diagnose particular medical problems would also be encouraged. Some CDHC enthusiasts even envision the development of a new kind of health care professional—the "health information counselor"—who would assist consumers in sifting through the vast amount of technical information that would be available. The hope is that this information would help people shop in the health care market as effectively and knowledgeably as they do in other service markets. The result would be more competition among health care providers, leading to lower costs and higher quality.

High-deductible insurance, HSAs, and more information for consumers are the three pillars of the CDHC plans now being tried in the health care marketplace, with the help of legislation passed by the Bush administration. But note that the legislation does not compel any changes in the behavior of private insurers. It simply encourages employers and consumers to choose high-deductible plans linked to HSAs. Neither does the legislation require any changes in the medical care delivery system. CDHC does not basically change the largely fee-for-service reimbursement of physicians, the itemized payment for outpatient technology, or the confusing and varied methods for hospital reimbursement used by the many different insurers. Nor does it mandate any change in the way health care is organized and delivered to patients. CDHC simply assumes that more individual participation in the health care market will bring about the desired reduction in costs and improvement in quality and convenience, without the need for more government intervention.

## The Business School Perspective

Some apostles of market-driven health care envision even more ex-
tensive reform. Prominent among these advocates is Regina Herzlinger, a Harvard Business School professor, who has been extolling
the virtues of a price-sensitive, consumer-driven, and competitive
health care market for many years. In the subtitle of her 1997 book
about CDHC, Herzlinger calls health care "America's largest service industry."[3] The reforms she proposes are predictable from
someone who believes health care is just another business, except
for the fact that she believes everyone under sixty-five should be required to buy high-deductible insurance of their choice and, if
needy, that they should receive subsidies from their employers or
from the government that are adjusted according to health status
and income. Otherwise, individuals should be on their own, as in
other markets. But full realization of consumer choice, she argues
in a more recent exposition of her views,[4] will require substantial
changes in the medical care delivery system that would make it
more like other competitive service industries.

She favors what she calls "focused factories," which means
groups of physicians and specialized facilities organized around the
delivery of a particular medical procedure or service, or the treatment of a particular ailment. She thinks this kind of segmentation
and specialization, much favored by business management experts
in other commercial markets, would promote competition and
help people choose just the services they want. Herzlinger believes
that "focused factories" would provide the most efficient and least
expensive treatment—assuming of course, that consumers' choices
are guided by readily available information about the competing
providers of the "focused" services. In extolling the virtues of "focused" care, she often cites the Shouldice Hospital in Ontario,
Canada, which does nothing but surgical repairs of simple hernias

in otherwise healthy people. I refer again to the Shouldice Hospital when I describe the Canadian health care system in Chapter 7.

Another prominent Harvard Business School professor, Michael Porter, has joined in the call for a more competitive, consumer-oriented health care system in a book written with Elizabeth Teisberg.[5] Like Herzlinger, Porter and Teisberg advocate competition at the level of individual services and individual physicians and facilities, but they believe quality (and outcome) is more important than price. They share with David Cutler the view that "increasing the value of the system," rather than simply using competition to force prices down, is the best way to deal with the cost crisis. They therefore advocate basing health care payments on quality, which would require the widest possible dissemination of information about the outcome of medical procedures and the performance of competing providers of care. In this respect, they align themselves with recent initiatives by government to make Medicare payments reflect the quality of the medical services being reimbursed ("payment for performance").[6]

Underlying the strategy of CDHC is the notion that health care, like other parts of the economy, is better left to individual decisions within the private sector than to government. People should be free to make their own choices about insurance and medical services because they know what they want and what they are willing to pay. According to this theory, individuals spending their own money in competitive markets for the services they want are the best means of getting the lowest prices and the highest quality. Government intervention can't achieve that. Its role should be confined to ensuring that competitive market forces are free to work their magic unimpeded by monopoly or fraud, that consumers have all the price and quality information they need, and that the poorest citizens are enabled (mainly through tax benefits) to participate as consumers in the medical marketplace.

The Bush administration likes to call its CDHC policies a part of "the ownership society," which it promotes as an antidote to "big government." It believes that private citizens—not government—should own and control more of our society's resources, including health care. What is not often mentioned, however, is that "ownership" of health care by private citizens also means that they, rather than government, pay for it. (They also "own" the bills.) The current administration evidently thinks that it is better to have citizens voluntarily pay out of pocket for their own health care than to tax them collectively to support government insurance. So, the Bush administration's enthusiasm for CDHC undoubtedly derives as much from its determination to reduce taxes—or, at least never raise them—as from its unshakable faith in a market-based solution for the rising costs of health care. As the current administration sees things, exempting HSAs and high-deductible health insurance premiums from taxes achieves a double purpose: It lowers taxes, and it encourages a private market in which individuals, rather than government, pay for health care.

## What's Wrong with the CDHC Proposals?

CDHC is a hot topic these days. Hardly a day passes without one or more articles in the popular media or health policy literature on consumerism, competition, HSAs, and high-deductible insurance policies. In the preceding pages I have summarized most of the arguments in support of a consumer-based market as the solution to the problems of rising costs, declining insurance coverage, and uneven quality. Now I will set out what I consider to be the most powerful arguments against CDHC, and the reasons I am convinced it will inevitably fail to achieve its stated goals.

*HSAs and high-deductible insurance plans are basically unfair because they will inevitably have the greatest impact on health services for the poor.* Low- and modest-income families would probably reduce their doctor visits and their use of routine and preventive medical services, so they wouldn't have to dip into their HSAs. That means that those with limited means, who most need the benefits of insurance coverage, would feel the greatest pressure not to seek care, while those who can more easily afford to pay the deductible would not hesitate to seek medical help. Preventive care, particularly immunizations, pediatric well-baby care, and routine visits for the care of chronic conditions in children and adults is likely to decline in a CDHC system—particularly among lower-income families needing to save money. Financial disincentives may reduce unnecessary visits to the doctor, but they also discourage many routine but necessary visits that may have serious long-term consequences for health.

Some advocates of high-deductible plans say this disproportionate effect on the poor could be avoided by adjusting the size of the deductible to income. But this is easier said than done. Assessments of ability to pay are difficult and would add greatly to administrative costs. A different approach has been suggested by the Bush administration, which favors tax credits as a way of equalizing the financial burdens of CDHC insurance, but this, too, is an untested idea. The fact remains that any attempt to curb overuse of health care resources by putting more financial responsibility on individual patients is bound to have a greater effect on the poor than the well-to-do.

Experience with current CDHC plans has been too brief and limited to justify the enthusiastic claims of their supporters, but the results of the much-touted RAND health insurance experiment (conducted from 1974 to 1982) are often cited as important empirical evidence that cost sharing by health care "consumers" can reduce national medical expenditures with no detrimental effects on health.[7] On close examination, however, the RAND study does not support such sweeping conclusions. The essential facts are that approximately 2,000 non-elderly families with low or middle incomes (mean income $30–$33,000 in 1991 dollars) were studied for three- or five-year periods while they were covered by different fee-for-service insurance plans designed by RAND, which provided comprehensive health care coverage with different levels of cost sharing. The cost sharing took the form of co-insurance, which ranged from 0 percent (that is, no co-payment by the beneficiary) to 95 percent (meaning the plan covered only 5 percent of charges). To persuade families to join the study, RAND had to guarantee "side payments" that would compensate for any financial loss sustained by switching from existing coverage to the experimental RAND plan. Health care expenditures during the three- or five-year period of observation and "health status" at the beginning and end of the experiment were measured and analyzed.

The results showed that despite the "side payments," there was a significant reduction in the use of all types of health care services in direct relation to the level of co-payment, amounting to a difference of about 25 to 30 percent in expenditures between the two extremes of cost sharing. Many commentators who cite this work seem to believe there were no significant differences in health outcome in any part of the population studied, but in fact, as the principal investigator, health economist Joseph Newhouse notes: "Health among the sick poor—approximately the most disadvantaged 6 percent of the population—was adversely affected. . . ."[8] The effects of reduced care in this group included higher mortality rates, less control of hypertension, poor eye care, and poor dental health. In short, the health of the poorest families suffered the most from cost sharing in this study—clear evidence of the basic unfairness of this approach to cost control.

In my judgment, those observed health care effects are made even more significant by the facts that follow-up was limited by the relatively brief duration of the study, the population studied was relatively young, and the methods of assessing health status were largely based on self-evaluation and relatively superficial physiological tests that could easily have overlooked serious underlying disease. Longer periods of study, older populations, and more thorough medical evaluation would probably have yielded larger effects on health status.

As for the impressive effect of cost sharing on the use of health care resources in this experiment, one needs to remember that the RAND investigators studied only subjects in families with low or modest incomes. Had they included families with larger incomes, the effects of co-payment on expenditures almost certainly would have been much less. It is a reasonable assumption that cost sharing would have less effect on families with higher incomes when they are deciding whether to seek medical help.

This consideration raises questions about the likelihood of CDHC (or co-payments, or any other kind of cost sharing) having much effect on total health expenditures when applied to an entire population. In fact, there is good reason to believe that cost sharing would not be nearly as effective in controlling total expenditures as claimed by its advocates. The major part of health expenditures is for serious disease and expensive procedures that involve a small part of the population. Health economists are generally agreed that the sickest 10 percent of the population accounts for about 70 percent of all expenditures.[9] Since high-deductible insurance plans would cover the majority of costs above the deductible and *all* costs beyond a specified out-of-pocket limit, such plans are not likely to reduce medical expenditures very much on those beneficiaries who use most of the expensive care. This conclusion is supported by the finding in the RAND experiment that levels of co-payment had no effect on the use of hospitalization for the treatment of serious illness. Most of the necessary big-ticket expenses were covered by insurance, regardless of deductibles or co-payment.

There is still another important reason that CDHC is not likely to control the rise of medical expenditures: It does not address the factors in the delivery system that are responsible for high and constantly rising costs. CDHC works primarily on the demand side of the health care economy by mitigating the moral hazard of first-dollar, low-deductible health insurance. Patients who have to pay more out of pocket for entrance into the medical care market are likely to be more cost sensitive—particularly if they have limited means. But increased use of expensive new technology contributes a large part of the health expenditure inflation, and this is driven mainly by factors on the supply side of the medical economy, which are unchanged by CDHC policies. New developments in medical science and technology, the rapid increase in the number of specialists whose practice depends on the use of new technology, the largely fee-for-service reimbursement of specialist physicians, the relatively high fees paid for technical procedures as opposed to cognitive services, and the intense market competition to increase revenues among institutions in the "medical-industrial complex" all contribute to rising expenditures by providing incentives to increase the supply of expensive services. None of these is changed by CDHC. Unless these supply-side factors are neutralized, control of rising medical expenses will continue to be almost impossible.

Not only would CDHC probably fail to control medical expenses, but it would also be very likely to undermine the entire system of insurance protection. Healthy young people would choose the least expensive plans with the highest allowable deductible, hoping to hold on to as much of their HSA as possible because it would be a form of tax-exempt savings. On the other hand, people with serious health problems, regardless of their income, would need to depend on insurance protection and would be forced to choose relatively expensive plans with the lowest allowable deductible. The premiums and the deductibles or the required co-payments on the latter plans would spiral upward because of the greater use of services by sicker beneficiaries, so it would become harder for those with the greatest need to afford coverage. The extent to which the CDHC system would lead to segmentation of the market between rich and poor, and healthy and sick, and to the exclusion of many poor sick families from the insurance market altogether is not yet known. Despite claims made by supporters that no such effects are occurring, it is much too soon to say. Nevertheless, one of the most important values of health insurance—the sharing of risks over a broad population base—would appear to be in serious jeopardy. Adjusting the HSA contribution from the employer or the government according to the health status of the beneficiaries has been suggested as a way of avoiding this problem, but the relatively primitive state of the art of "risk adjustment" and the difficulty in applying it to whole families make this solution unlikely and would add greatly to administrative costs.

What about effects of CDHC on the quality of medical care? Contrary to the claims of its advocates, CDHC would impede efforts to improve the functions of the medical care delivery system. One of the basic requirements for improvement of medical care is that physicians and health care facilities work together—or at least cooperate—in the care of each patient. That is what the Institute of Medicine called for in its 2001 report,[10] but none of its recommendations could be implemented if medical consumers went shopping from provider to provider in a competitive marketplace, looking for the services they wanted at the prices they were willing to pay—in effect acting as their own primary care physician.

Neither could there be much general improvement in the quality of care if doctors and hospitals functioned as independent vendors do in ordinary service markets, simply responding to the demands of consumers. The important tasks of evaluating and interpreting symptoms, of coordinating and integrating services for each patient, and of deciding which specialty services and which institutions and facilities would best meet the needs of each patient would be left to the patients themselves. Most patients would be daunted by such responsibility and few could take it on. Despite all the new information sources that might be available to consumers, this is a task that requires the professional knowledge of a physician.

Another problem with CDHC concerns the keeping of medical records. Who would keep the patient's medical record? Few patients would have the medical background to even understand, let alone manage, their medical records. Very likely each physician and hospital would keep their own, and records would continue to be separated. There would be no place for an integrated and complete medical record. It is hard to imagine how modern information technology (the electronic record) could be used and who would pay for it, if patients were expected to act as independent consumers of medical services without the benefit of professional supervision and coordination of their care. Electronic medical records have been successfully adopted only within institutions or organizations where physicians practice together under unified management, such as large group practices or the VA medical system. It is unlikely that this kind of clinical advance could be adopted (and paid for) by the large numbers of unorganized independent practitioners who now provide most of the medical care in our current system.

As for the "focused factory" idea championed by Herzlinger, that is a delusion born of unfamiliarity with the realities of medical care. True, some specific treatments and procedures could be (and are) provided by independent groups and facilities that more or less exclusively focus on one kind of service. (Examples are centers for imaging or kidney dialysis, and hospitals that specialize in one type of treatment such as Canada's Shouldice Hospital for hernia surgery, or U.S. investor-owned hospitals that specialize in cardiovascular or orthopedic surgery.) But few physicians would believe that our health care system could be entirely or even largely based on hundreds or thousands of independent, competing physician groups and medical facilities that specialized in only one particular disease or ailment, as proposed by the advocates of "focused factories." Patients often suffer from multiple ailments simultaneously or develop additional ailments over time and therefore need help from many specialists and many kinds of technology. When patients are treated for a serious problem with one organ or organ system, they often develop other complications involving other organs. For each "focused factory" to have available all the other specialists and facilities that might be needed to deal with those problems makes no sense at all and would be wasteful of resources.[11]

The idea of "focused factories," which envisions specialized independent facilities, should be distinguished from an internal arrangement that is commonly found in large general hospitals, where a particular area may be devoted to the treatment of a particular disease or group of diseases, or where a particular type of surgical care is concentrated. This kind of localization of personnel and equipment is efficient but requires that other resources, specialists, and consultants be available within the same institution to deal with complications or with other coexisting diseases.

Medical care under a fully developed CDHC system (including "focused factories") would be fragmented and chaotic, to say the least. Continuity of care would be nonexistent, unless the patient took on that responsibility. And that would be very unlikely to improve the quality—or the efficiency—of the care. More likely, the quality of care would deteriorate as patients tried to act as their own physicians, seeking to find their way as inexpensively as possible through a bewildering medical marketplace, amid a confusion of competing advertising claims.

The theory of CDHC envisions that patients' decisions would be supported by a greatly improved system of readily available information. While I have no doubt that there are many ways by which more reliable and useful information about the costs and quality of health insurance plans, health care providers, and health care facilities could be distributed to the public, I do not believe such information could replace the need for expert advice from physicians. Nor could it provide essential information about each individual's health status. As "consumers," patients may be able to make good use of public information in choosing insurance plans, physicians, and hospitals, but even under the best of circumstances they cannot be expected to act as their own physicians in deciding whether they are ill, what is wrong, and what ought to be done. And when they are seriously ill or injured, people are even less able to manage their own health care. Physicians who themselves have been seriously injured or sick know that lesson very well. When they are in trouble, they seek the best medical advice they can get and do not attempt independently to diagnose or treat themselves.

This is not to say that patients should not be as fully informed about their health problems as they wish, and as they realistically can be. To the greatest extent possible, and to the degree they desire, patients should participate with their physicians in making the decisions about how they are treated. In today's health care system, whether they are insured or not, they certainly should have access to information about treatment options and their costs. But if they are sensible, they will want the advice of a capable and caring physician in deciding on how to proceed and what interventions are safe and worthwhile. "Consumer-driven health care" is a catchy phrase, but it is an illusion that bears little resemblance to the realities when seriously sick or injured patients turn to the health care system for help. Those who confidently assert the ability of the informed consumer to choose his or her own medical care in that situation usually have not been seriously injured or sick themselves. There are very few prudent shoppers in hospital emergency rooms or intensive care units, and no bargain hunters in cancer clinics.

There is one final consideration that should make anyone genuinely interested in improving our health care system pause before endorsing CDHC and, in particular, the concept of HSAs. If HSAs grow as predicted over the next few years, they will constitute a huge new source of tax-exempt private savings that will bring the financial management industry into the health care system. An article in the *New York Times* on January 27, 2006, headed "Health Savings Accounts Attract Wall St.," described how "Banks, credit unions and money management firms are now quietly positioning themselves to become central players in the business of health care. . . ." The article went on to say: "Not since the creation of the individual retirement account in the mid-1970s has such a potentially huge mountain of money landed in the lap of the financial services industry." This money will be invested in stocks, bonds, and mutual funds under the direction of financial companies, which of course profit from management fees and earned interest. Even the insurance companies selling the high-deductible plans are setting up their own banks to cash in on this new business opportunity. Financial institutions, formerly uninterested in health care policy, now lobby the Bush administration in support of CDHC and urge expansion of the tax benefits for HSAs.

So HSAs will be another opportunity for the health care system in the United States to become a financial playground for investors and investor-owned businesses. Here is another way in which money that ought to be paying for health care will be siphoned off for other purposes. This result of CDHC is yet another demonstration that treating health care as a market adds to administrative and management costs and puts influence over policy decisions in the hands of those whose primary business is money and not health care.

In summary, I believe CDHC plans are unrealistic and unfair, and I doubt they will prove to be acceptable in the long run. While I believe individuals should have at least some responsibility for the cost of purely elective or optional medical services, I join with the majority of U.S. citizens who think that the availability of needed medical services should not depend on the ability to pay. We are an advanced, wealthy society, and decency requires that we make equitable arrangements to ensure at least minimally adequate health care for all—a goal that would be lost under CDHC, or any other system that relies on market forces to distribute care. Beyond its glaring inequity, however, CDHC suffers from a fundamental misconception that makes it unlikely to control rising costs. The concept of the patient as a consumer in a medical marketplace is deeply flawed. It is unlikely that consumer choices, even if given greater play, would significantly moderate the inflation of medical expenditures.

CDHC plans of one kind or another are nevertheless firmly embedded in current thinking about health policy and will surely be more widely tested in both the public and private insurance sectors. So strong is the current belief in market-based policy such as CDHC, and so powerful are the economic interests profiting from the commercialization of our health care system, that it will take considerable time—at least, I would guess, another decade—before a major change in the direction of national health policy becomes feasible. Substantial reform will probably have to wait for CDHC to play itself out, just as investor-owned "managed care" and HMOs did over the last few years. In the course of this "playing out," the system is likely to become so dysfunctional, and its costs so onerous, that the availability of services to the poor will decline even more, the number of uninsured and underinsured will continue to grow, and the scandalous inequity between the care of the rich and the poor will become unacceptable. At that juncture, public opinion—joined, I hope by the large part of the business community that pays for health care, and by most of the medical profession—will demand major reform.

# 5

# THE REFORM WE NEED

> The problems in the U.S. are systemic. Incremental changes cannot solve them; further reliance on market-based strategies will exacerbate them. What needs to be changed is the system itself. . . . A national health insurance program is the only affordable option for universal, comprehensive coverage.
>
> —PHYSICIANS' WORKING GROUP FOR SINGLE-PAYER NATIONAL HEALTH INSURANCE, *JAMA*, 2003

IF THE MARKET IS NOT GOING TO SAVE OUR HEALTH CARE SYSTEM, must we conclude that the system's problems are intractable? Must we settle for marginal, incremental improvements and hope that the system somehow manages to survive? Many health policy experts seem to think so. The Commonwealth Fund has been conducting polls among these experts that suggest that the experts have a different assessment of health care problems than the one I present in this book. "Expansion of coverage to the uninsured" and "increased use of information technology to improve the quality and safety of care" are given higher priority for congressional action than "reforms to moderate the rising costs of medical care." And, among the possible approaches to achieving cost control, improved information technology and payment incentives to providers for quality and efficiency are given the highest priority.

The respondents to the Commonwealth polls appear to overlook major reform of the insurance or the delivery sectors of health care in favor of more limited, technical improvements in the system we have. That seems to agree with the present prevailing wisdom of all those authorities who, regardless of their opinion about "consumer-driven health care," reject the possibility of major reform. Some might "in principle" favor major reform, but probably regard it as utopian and unrealistic. They therefore take the position held by most health economists, and advocate more conservative, piecemeal improvements.

I reject such an approach because I do not agree it is our only practical choice. Furthermore, the suggested piecemeal improvements do not directly address the underlying problems of our health care system, which are likely to continue to plague us unless we finally resolve them with stronger measures. I regard the policies currently favored by most experts as inadequate responses to an approaching crisis that threatens to undermine the system within the next decade or so. Most of these proposals either increase costs or reduce coverage and quality. I am convinced that a more satisfactory solution is possible, but only with major reform.

It is neither possible nor desirable at this juncture to offer more than a broad strategy. Most of the details of a workable plan, and perhaps even some of its basic foundations, will have to be drawn up in the future, as circumstances dictate. But we need to start the discussion and planning process now. My purpose here is simply to demonstrate that a practical, workable solution is possible, and that we as a nation can achieve an affordable, good quality, and equitable health care system—if we really want it.

The plan I propose draws in part on an earlier proposal published by the Physicians' Working Group for Single-Payer National Insurance,[1] but goes beyond it by suggesting major reform of the medical care delivery system as well. Any reformed system that stands a chance of controlling costs, while still providing universal coverage and improving the quality of care, must change not only the present insurance system but also the organization and style of medical practice. This is my major difference with the physicians' proposal, which focuses mainly on achieving a single-payer insurance system. I believe single-payer insurance is necessary, but it will not control costs sufficiently unless we also reform the way physicians are organized in practice and how they are paid.[2]

## Funding and Insurance

Consider first the funding of the health care system. Lack of money is not our problem. We currently spend a little over *$2 trillion per year* on health care. That amounts to some $7,000 per man, woman, and child, healthy or sick—or roughly $25,000 annually for the average family. For that kind of money, as any experienced health insurance actuary will tell you, we ought to be able to obtain universal coverage and good-quality care for all. So why haven't we had those benefits? It is because a large proportion of what we spend is directed toward profits and unnecessary overhead, and management and business expenses (including marketing and advertising), or is wasted on unneeded or ineffective medical procedures, or is lost to fraud and abuse in billing practices. No one has any hard data on the total cost of all this diversion of resources from health care to other ends, but my best guess is that it represents at least one-third of our total health care expenditures, and quite possibly as much as 40 to 45 percent. That is an enormous and continuously growing sum, which would be much better spent on providing universal coverage and improving the quality of care. A reformed system that eliminated most or all of this diversion would probably not need any more money to achieve its goals—at least not in the beginning. We would need only to sustain the present level of funding.

A dysfunctional, high-overhead insurance system accounts for an important part of this diversion of resources, and almost all of the insurance overhead is in the private sector of the system. A major difficulty with private insurance is that it is splintered into many hundreds of competing plans, the great majority of which are investor-owned businesses. There are, of course, many not-for-profit private insurance plans, but collectively they probably cover less than one-fourth of all privately insured patients. For-profit insurance businesses extract their profits and their overhead and management costs from the premium before paying doctors and hospitals for services provided. This amounts to a diversion of approximately 10 to 25 percent of the premium. By comparison, the overhead costs of private not-for-profit plans are about half that amount. *I can find no evidence that the for-profit plans add anything that is worth this extra cost.*

The higher overhead cost of investor-owned insurance is probably due largely to profits, marketing, more expensive management, and the cost of the more aggressive underwriting (that is, adjusting premiums according to health risks of the insured) and the screening needed to avoid high-risk groups. Insurance companies make money when their customers are healthy and do not need medical services. They are at risk when they insure beneficiaries who are chronically ill or likely to become ill. To protect against such risks, many investor-owned plans adjust their premiums according to the health of their beneficiaries, or by various means simply avoid insuring risky groups. All of these practices add to the insurers' expenses, and to offset these extra costs, private insurers must make money from investments, raise premiums, or reduce benefits. The overhead costs of public insurance plans such as Medicare (about 3 percent) are much lower than even those of private not-for-profit plans.

In addition to the overhead costs that insurers must bear, there are the expenses providers of medical care face in dealing with the administrative requirements of multiple insurance plans—public as well as private. To receive payment, physicians, hospitals, and all institutions providing care spend large amounts of money on personnel and office facilities devoted to meeting the diverse regulations of multiple insurers. Private practice office staffs as well as the business departments of hospitals have grown enormously to deal with billing transactions involving multiple payers. Large hospitals must now employ literally hundreds of people to handle the tasks of billing and collecting from many different insurers. Physicians in private practice must spend time on the phone with insurers to explain their bills and respond to requests for more information. Furthermore, the enormously complicated procedure of billing and collecting provides innumerable opportunities for inflating charges and for outright fraud—which siphons away an estimated 5 to 10 percent of medical expenditures in some regions and some parts of the system.

Conceivably, market competition among private health plans in a "consumer-driven" system might mitigate some of these problems. But this would require that plans be persuaded or legally mandated to disclose all the relevant information about their payment and management practices, prices, and benefits. Even in that unlikely event, most of the insurance problems described above would still remain. Clearly the best and most definitive solution would be to replace the present fragmented, inefficient, and expensive insurance system with a relatively simplified single-payer plan that would eliminate the present hassle, expense, and complexity of billing and collecting for services.

## A Workable "Single-Payer" Insurance Plan

The term "single payer" can be used to describe a variety of health care systems that have one common feature: Doctors and hospitals and other direct providers of care are paid through a single agency, rather than through the multiplicity of payers characteristic of our present health care system. The central payment agency could receive its funds from one or multiple sources (for example, government, employers, or individuals) and could pay health care providers in various ways. The organization of the medical care delivery system could take many different forms under a single-payer plan, and the single-payer agency itself could be administered by government, by a private non-profit organization under government licensure, or by some type of combined public-private arrangement.

The single-payer insurance system I favor would be supported by a health care fund, generated from an earmarked health care tax levied by Congress at graduated rates based on income or assets, and it would cover everyone. Government would pay into the fund for those with little or no income or assets. The actual rate of the health care tax would be legislatively adjusted, perhaps biennially, to ensure receipts large enough to meet all anticipated needs of the health care system. This would also provide an effective means for capping costs. The Physicians' Working Group envisions the funds supporting the system arising from a variety of sources, including existing taxes, but I believe a separate, earmarked health care tax would be essential in order to keep the financing of health care totally away from the volatility of the annual budgetary process in Congress.

At the start of the plan, the health care taxes that would otherwise be levied on the former beneficiaries of private plans (that is, employees) could be offset by appropriate payments to the health care fund from employers. These payments would approximate the amount previously contributed by employers to their employees' insurance, so employers would not be asked to contribute more than they did under the old system. Eventually, the employers' obligations might be phased out by increases in wages sufficient for employees to pay their own health tax, thus breaking the unnatural and dysfunctional connection between employment and health insurance. The government's obligation to cover the cost of health insurance for the poor, the disabled, and the elderly should continue under any single-payer insurance plan. Medicaid and Medicare would be subsumed in the new insurance plan, and all those covered by those programs would have their health care tax paid by government, as would the uninsured poor. Coverage would be universal, and there would be no loss of present federal and state benefits.

We do not need more money to reform the system as described here. Rather, we need to find a way to pool all our current health care payments and use them to fund a more efficient system that would avoid most of the expenditures now wasted on excessive overhead and management costs, profits, fraud, and overuse of expensive technology, procedures, and drugs.

Like the Physicians' Working Group, I believe everyone should be guaranteed all the health care benefits prescribed by their physicians, including ambulatory and inpatient services, acute and long-term care, and drugs, psychiatric care, and home care. Dental services would also be covered. The only exclusions from benefits would be certain services listed by a national advisory board as not medically necessary or ineffective, or outside the accepted boundaries of needed medical care, such as most elective aesthetic plastic surgery and cosmetic procedures, private hospital rooms and nurses, and most varieties of "alternative" therapies that have not been proven effective in clinical trials. The list of excluded services would be under continuous review, in response to emerging evidence about safety and effectiveness.

To be successful, a national insurance plan must meet the needs and expectations of very nearly the entire population. Nevertheless, in U.S. society patients will want choices. Those desiring services *not* covered under the national plan should be able to obtain them outside the system (that is, provided by health professionals who are not part of the plan), but at their own expense or through privately purchased insurance. They should also be able to obtain services outside the national system that *are* covered by the plan, but only through direct personal payment. No private insurance should be allowed to compete with the national plan by selling coverage of services available through the plan, and no resources from the plan should be used to pay for services delivered outside the system, whether or not they are available through the national plan.

Because virtually all insured services would be reimbursed on a prepaid, per capita basis (see below), there would be no billing or payment transactions. The Physicians' Working Group would allow physicians working in the national plan to choose fee-for-service reimbursement if they wished, but this I believe would generate cost control problems that my proposal would avoid. I think fee-for-service payment should be totally eliminated from the national plan. Instead, I favor requiring all physicians working in the plan to be salaried by prepaid medical groups, or to be on the salaried staff of a hospital or other certified facility. Salaries might be supplemented by modest bonuses, as determined by the management of a prepaid multi-specialty group practice (PGP; see below) or hospital, but the total payment to all the physicians on a PGP or hospital staff would be limited by regulation. In the plan I envision, PGPs would keep a record of all services rendered, and these could be electronically reported to central agencies in cumulative, depersonalized forms as needed. PGPs would not submit bills to the central insurance agency, and there would be no piecework payment to them. This would save the huge overhead costs of billing transactions and would eliminate opportunities for billing fraud.

Should patients pay anything for services as they are provided? The Physicians' Working Group says no, but there are reasonable arguments pro and con about such "user fees." Therefore, I suggest that this be one of the questions that might be deferred for later resolution, based perhaps on initial experience with the system. These fees, or co-payments, do reduce the use of many services, as the RAND insurance experiment demonstrated, but the long-term health consequences of such reductions are troubling. How effectively the reformed medical care delivery system proposed below could prevent overuse of services, and thus avoid the need for co-payments, remains to be seen.

## A Reformed Medical Care Delivery System

Payment for comprehensive health care services on a prepaid per capita basis would greatly simplify national budgetary planning and would avoid most of the overhead costs. But to control the rise in its expenditures and assure quality of care, such a payment system would require a new kind of medical care delivery system that could optimally allocate the capitated (annual per person) payment and manage medical resources. Effective deployment of medical resources requires expert knowledge of when and how to treat patients. Physicians are better qualified than government, employers, insurance plans, or patients to assume this responsibility, but they must be organized in a way that allows them to use their best judgment, uninfluenced by financial incentives or constraints that prevent them from meeting their professional commitment to patients.

The medical organization best suited to that purpose is the prepaid multi-specialty group practice (PGP).[3] These are teams of physicians, including primary care doctors as well as specialists, who practice together with nurses and other health professionals in one or more common facilities and provide comprehensive care for an prearranged annual per person payment. My proposal for a single-payer prepaid insurance system therefore calls for replacement of private solo practices and small single-specialty partnerships with community-based multi-specialty PGPs. Some well-known, successful examples of PGPs include such giants as Kaiser-Permanente, Group Health of Puget Sound, and Harvard-Vanguard. They are, in effect, staff- or group-model HMOs, because they provide prepaid health insurance as well as an organized system that delivers medical care. The primary care physicians in these systems are usually paid a salary, variably supplemented with bonuses. Specialists are paid variously.

At present, there are a few hundred multi-specialty group practices in the country, but most are not prepaid and do not also market their own insurance plan. They provide care on an episodic fee-for-service basis, receiving payment from many different independent insurance plans. A few large multi-specialty fee-for-service group practices, including the Mayo Clinic, the Marshfield Clinic (Wisconsin) and the Scott & White Clinic (Texas), also market their own insurance programs and function both as a PGP and an HMO for some of the patients they serve. The Physicians' Working Group would have PGPs as one practice option that physicians might choose, but I believe a single-payer insurance system would work much better if most practicing physicians either were members of smaller, community-based PGPs or were on the salaried staff of certified hospitals or other certified facilities. Independent private practice should be the choice of relatively few, who would be outside the national plan.

The medical care system I envision would be primarily based on PGPs of approximately 50 to 100 physicians, about half of whom would be primary care doctors and the remainder of whom would be specialists. Staffing by physicians would be supplemented by nurse practitioners and physicians' assistants, so the number of physicians in a group might vary considerably. All groups would be certified by a new national agency, created by legislative action and accountable to Congress (see below, under Management of the System). To be certified, each group would have enough primary care physicians and specialists to provide good care for the number of patients they would be permitted to enroll. As an example, the average 100-physician group with 50 primary care physicians might be expected to enroll a maximum of 75,000 patients, thus allowing no more than 1,500 patients per primary care physician (supported by nurse practitioners and physicians' assistants). In less densely populated areas, smaller groups would enroll proportionately fewer patients. Rural areas could be served by small teams of community-based physicians and nurses who would be affiliated with a PGP in a nearby larger population center. Given modern communication and transportation, there is no reason why all but the most remote regions of the country could not be covered by physicians and related professional personnel working as part of a more centrally located multi-specialty PGP. In this way, residents in virtually all of the country could have the benefits of medical care from a group practice, and physicians would have the widest choice of geographic location for their practice.

Each certified PGP would be privately managed as a not-for-profit professional partnership. It would be expected to provide all the ambulatory services covered by the central insurance plan and, within broad guidelines, be free to recruit its own professional and administrative personnel. The physicians in the group would be paid from a pool of money that would be a defined percentage of the total capitated insurance funds received from the central payer. Presumably, that percentage (determined by the central agency) would be close to the fraction of personal health expenditures that currently remains with physicians as net income in our present system. At present, practicing physicians retain about 10 to 12 percent of their gross practice income, after paying the cost of their practice expenses and their fringe benefits. Since all of these latter costs would be covered by the group, the earmarked 10 to 12 percent would be paid to physicians by their PGP mainly as salaries, probably supplemented by bonuses, as determined by the elected medical management of the group. Although privately managed, each group would be publicly accountable for its management and for the quality of its services. Groups would be expected to use standardized electronic information technology (IT), so that all data, with privacy appropriately protected, could be integrated into a national reporting system. The benefits derived from such a standardized and integrated IT system would be immense, but such a system is almost impossible to develop in our present health care system.

There would be no place in the system for profits, and the PGPs would be no exception. As not-for-profit community-service institutions, the groups would be protected against losses due to adverse selection or to other costs beyond their control.[4] They would receive help with start-up expenses and capital costs (including information technology) and would be exempt from antitrust regulation. Such exemption would require legislation that would define certified groups as not being engaged in interstate commerce and therefore not subject to antitrust laws. Any operating net revenue would not accrue to physicians or administrators but could only be used to improve services and facilities. Administrative salaries, like physician income, would be established by each group's executive committee under guidelines set by the governing national agency. Groups would compete for patients on the basis of the quality of their services and their reputation in the community. There would be no price competition because all patients would have the same benefits and would not have to pay for individual services as received.

All groups would be open to all citizens, although the number of members per group would be limited to ensure an appropriate ratio of doctors to patients. Patients would be free to choose their own group, as well as the physicians they wanted within the group, and to change their group membership at any time. Patients would also be free to seek care within the universal plan from a specialist who was outside their particular group but still a member of the plan. If they wanted services outside the plan or not covered by it, they would have to consult a physician who was outside the plan and pay out of pocket. However, everyone would have to be a member of some group, just as they would have to pay their health care tax (or have the government or their employer pay it for them). In a universal system like this, these rules should also apply to government officials and legislators, because they would be unlikely to neglect the support of a system that provided all or most of the care for themselves and their families.

Physicians would be free to join any group or become a salaried member of any facility that wished to hire them, and to change that affiliation under mutually agreed terms. They would also be free to practice entirely outside the plan, but they could not then be paid for their services by the plan. I do not think physicians should be allowed to divide their practice time between the plan and independent practice—they should have to choose one or the other. Otherwise, the public plan might well be neglected by some physicians who would have access to wealthy patients but could also benefit from seeing other patients within the plan if they wished. To protect its quality, the public system has to be supported well enough to meet the expectations of the great majority of physicians, who would be committed to making it work well.

## Health Care Facilities

In addition to the groups, which would provide most of the insured ambulatory services, medical care would be delivered by a network of other ambulatory care facilities, hospitals, long-term care institutions, and diagnostic facilities similar to those now existing in our health care system. They would all be not-for-profit and would get most of their patients through referral from the physicians in the groups. However, teaching hospitals, especially those that are part of academic health centers, might also wish to form their own group practices and generate some of their own referrals. In any case, they could hire physicians who would devote all of their practice time to providing services on their staff or who might divide their practice time between a PGP and one or more facility.

How should all these other facilities be paid? The plan proposed by the Physicians' Working Group suggests negotiated global budgets from the regional office of the central payer, with separate budgets for operating and capital expenses. This would be similar to the way hospitals are budgeted in Canada, except that each Canadian province is independently responsible for funding its own hospitals rather than having hospital budgets negotiated by a national agency, as proposed by the Physicians' Working Group in the U.S. plan. Although good arguments can be made in support of the Physicians' Working Group proposal, I believe it would be better if hospitals and other facilities submitted bills to PGPs for services they rendered to the group's patients and had to compete for referrals on the basis of the quality of their service—but not on the basis of prices. The physicians in the PGPs (and their patients) would be the best judges of quality, and competition among facilities would be a strong incentive to provide good services. Global budgeting from a central insurer eliminates this incentive and adds administrative complexity that increases the health system's overhead.

I agree with the Physicians' Working Group that all facilities should be not-for-profit, like the PGPs. Furthermore, their prices should be regulated and fully disclosed so there could be no special dealing between facilities and PGPs. Like the PGPs, facilities should be protected against the financial risks of treating very sick or complicated patients. This would remove any incentives to underserve patients and would help to ensure optimum treatment for all.

Although I believe short-term facilities would probably fare better if they were paid for services rendered to each patient, global budgeting might be more appropriate for long-term facilities such as nursing homes and rehabilitation facilities. These facilities are normally not paid on an itemized basis and could easily adapt to a budget negotiated with the central payer.

Converting all facilities to not-for-profit status is a major problem that will require careful planning. I cannot suggest in detail how this should be accomplished, but I assume that investors and owners would be fairly compensated from the central health fund for the value of their equity at the time of the transition. Those for-profit facilities deemed important enough to preserve would be transferred for their management to local not-for-profit boards appointed by regional representatives of the central health agency. These arrangements would be established through legislation, but I would guess that at least some of these transfers would be accomplished through private deals in which existing not-for-profit facilities merged with their for-profit competition.

Teaching hospitals need special mention here because in addition to offering the usual services to patients, they educate medical students, nurses, house officers, and clinical fellows, do a large share of the clinical research on new drugs, devices, and procedures, and serve as referral centers for specialized care and cutting-edge medical technology that would not be available in the usual community hospital. To carry out these essential functions, teaching hospitals need larger professional and technical staffs and more elaborate facilities than nonteaching hospitals of similar size, and they need extra funding. Medicare payments to teaching hospitals currently include a subsidy for this purpose, but it is inadequate and always vulnerable to reductions as part of the annual congressional budget-setting process. Medicaid payments often don't even meet costs of routine care, and they are grossly inadequate compensation for the extra costs of teaching hospitals. The need to cross-subsidize these costs has tempted too many teaching hospitals to look for income from joint ventures with the drug, biotech, and medical device industries. These may compromise the hospitals' integrity as not-for-profit academic institutions.

Whatever payment method is chosen for hospital care in a reformed system, teaching hospitals should receive adequate and predictable support from the central payment agency or the regional authority for their special functions, and the necessary funds should be held apart from the mainstream financing of the health care system. The cost of this payment would be a very small fraction of the total disbursements from the health care fund, probably less than 5 percent, and would be easily affordable. In a reformed system, we should be able to stabilize the finances of our teaching hospitals and protect their professional independence.

## Management of the System

The health care fund and the general administration and coordination of the medical care system should be in the hands of a new agency—let us call it here the National Medical Care Agency (NMCA). It would be created by legislative action and be accountable to Congress, but it should have independent and stable authority, which would protect it from variable political winds in the legislative and executive branches of government. It should be directed by a relatively small group of recognized experts in the field, to be nominated by the important organizations and constituencies in health care and appointed for long, rotating terms by the president. The directors would be supported by a large staff of professionals and administrators who would carry out the work and maintain appropriate records. In many respects, the NMCA would resemble such agencies as the Securities and Exchange Commission, the Federal Trade Commission, and the Federal Reserve Board, which are invested with independent authority to regulate important sectors of our economy. Since so much of health care is local, the NMCA should be decentralized to a considerable degree. It would have offices in every state or every region, to oversee all the local health care organizations and activities and work with all the local agencies affected by the reorganized health care system.

The NMCA would necessarily be a relatively large government organization, with a significant budget derived from the revenues of the health care tax. But it would be replacing a huge network of existing federal and state agencies, so the net result would probably be a substantial savings in administrative expense. The new universal health care insurance system would be much simpler than the current mishmash of competing and overlapping public and private plans, so it seems likely that its administrative costs would also be much less. Nevertheless, those who design the new system would need to take great care to avoid the temptation of an overly complex administrative organization. That was one of the major flaws in the ill-fated Clinton proposals of 1993.

The major function of the NMCA would be to regulate and oversee the operation of the health care system. It would not deal directly with, or employ, doctors, nurses, or other health care personnel. They would be employed by the private groups, hospitals, and various facilities involved in the delivery of care. Neither would the NMCA own any facilities. In short, the system could not be described as "socialized medicine." That term means government ownership of facilities and government employment of the personnel delivering the care. The system I envision would consist largely of privately owned not-for-profit institutions and a private workforce hired by those institutions. Physicians within the system would be responsible for their own management, although they would all be working within an organization that was supported by tax funds and regulated by a single public-private agency.

The NMCA would also be responsible for defining the services and goods that could not be covered by the national plan; but within that framework, the deployment of the services that were covered would be determined by the physicians caring for the patients in each group practice. The NMCA would be responsible for certifying the physician groups and health care facilities that are eligible to participate in the plan. Goods prescribed or used by the physicians in the groups, including prescription drugs and medical devices, would not be selected by the NMCA, nor would the NMCA decide how or when they should be used—that would also be the responsibility of the physician groups—but the NMCA would negotiate prices with the manufacturers.

## Would a Reformed System
## Solve Today's Problems?

The major problems facing our current system are control of medical costs, finding the resources to fund those costs, providing universal coverage, and ensuring the quality and accessibility of care. At the beginning of this book, I explained why the cost problem must be solved if we are to afford universal coverage. The reform plan I have outlined in this chapter would not only control costs but would help to achieve the other goals as well. It would control and fund health care expenditures in a simple and direct manner. Each year—or, better, every two years—Congress would establish a total national budget for health care, which would be closely linked to the expected revenues from the health care tax and would reflect a publicly determined decision on how much the nation wants to spend. The allocation of the national health care budget among the various categories of health-related functions would be a prime responsibility of NMCA. Most of the budget assigned to personal health care services would be distributed on an adjusted per capita basis to the medical groups, which would be responsible for directing the internal expenditure of those resources for the comprehensive care of their members, including the cost of prescription drugs and the cost of caring for patients in hospital facilities.

The size of the per capita payment distributed to the medical groups would be inversely related to the allocations for other covered health care personal services such as long-term care, dental services, mental health, community services, and so on. The part of the total budget not allocated to personal health service, such as expenditures for education, clinical research, and construction costs, might require different types of oversight. In any case, the total cost of administering the national health care budget would almost certainly be less than the present huge overhead costs of today's fragmented and heavily commercialized insurance and medical care delivery systems. In contrast to our present situation, the system envisioned here would have a clearly defined and controllable total cost, and an equally clearly defined and controllable source of funds, that is, the health care tax. Administrative and overhead savings in the insurance and delivery sectors of the reformed system described here would be substantial.

An equal, perhaps even greater, source of savings in the new system would stem from the change in the style of medical practice and the incentives of physician and institutional providers. Physicians practicing in not-for-profit groups that are paid on a capitated basis would have much less incentive to over- or underuse resources than in a fee-for-service private practice system. They would more likely employ technology according to accepted standards and professional on-the-ground judgment and be much less influenced by entrepreneurial motives. Drugs would be prescribed in a more rational and conservative manner, based more on published clinical studies and less on marketing hype. Physicians in well-managed multi-specialty groups tend to adhere to standards that are monitored by their own internal peer-review procedures; the result is a more prudent, evidence-based practice style that is also less costly. Elimination of the investor ownership of hospitals and ambulatory facilities would reduce the incentives for these facilities to market their services. And reduced marketing would certainly help to control rising expenditures.

The system outlined here could achieve universal coverage without adding costs. The combined savings from the insurance and the medical care delivery sectors could easily amount to at least 30 percent of present expenses. That would be more than enough to pay the costs of covering all those now uninsured, and to reduce or eliminate the need for most, if not all, out-of-pocket contributions from beneficiaries. To afford universal coverage, we must first develop a new system that lowers costs and controls inflation without impairing the quality of care.

Adoption of the reforms suggested here would also greatly improve the quality of medical care. The quality of any modern medical care system is shaped by the way physicians practice, and the best medical care can be realized when physicians practice in organized teams, where incentives for competent service and cooperation with other health care professionals are more important than the entrepreneurial incentives of fee-for-service private practice. Service on a state licensing and disciplinary board taught me that it is usually solo practitioners, not members of organized groups, who are most likely to face disciplinary action—probably because informal peer review in group practices deals with substandard practitioners before they get in trouble. Lacking any day-to-day professional oversight, solo practitioners can more easily go astray. Furthermore, without the financial support of a group, practitioners are more likely to feel economic pressures that may cause them to neglect medical standards, as they strive for greater income.

A growing problem with today's commercialized and competitive medical care system is the insidious erosion of professional norms and their replacement by business values. As investors become an ever-larger part of the system and physicians are encouraged—or forced by economic circumstances—to regard their practice as a business, the ethical principles of the medical profession are forgotten. Physicians perform their best when they truly believe that the welfare of their patients is their greatest responsibility, but in today's climate that belief is more of a public relations mantra than a guide for action. The reforms proposed here would help physicians regain their ethical balance. Properly organized and motivated, they should be better able to serve their patients, while finding greater satisfaction in their profession.

# 6

---

# CAN WE GET THERE?
# DO WE WANT TO?

> It is an issue of will and commitment. At some point
> we as a nation will have to decide whether we wish to
> design our health care system primarily to satisfy those
> who profit from it or to protect the health and welfare
> of all Americans.
>
> —DAVID MECHANIC, *THE TRUTH*
> *ABOUT HEALTH CARE*, 2006

TO ORGANIZE AND IMPLEMENT THE CHANGES NECESSARY TO
reshape our health care system would be a large public undertak-
ing. Given the magnitude and complexity of the task, and the political opposition it would have to overcome, a reform of this kind
would appear to be virtually impossible—at least for the immediate future.

Indeed, that is the consensus of most expert observers today. Instead of major reform, the health care pundits expect continuing
and expanded efforts to bring market forces into play, such as
CDHC. Most also advocate limited government initiatives to ame-
liorate some of the most pressing problems of the poor and uninsured. Few acknowledge the need for the kind of basic reform I
advocate—a single-payer universal insurance system and a reorganized, non-profit system for delivering care—and almost no one

thinks such reform has a chance of being seriously considered by Congress right now.

Remember, however, that most of these skeptical experts are trained in economics, a discipline that favors free markets and distrusts government regulation. Although a few prominent health economists have reservations, the great majority are convinced that market forces can ultimately resolve our health care problems, and they would certainly oppose the kind of reform advocated here. Many lawmakers share these views and pay close attention to the economists' advice.

Supporting and encouraging the opinions of the health economists and the market-oriented lawmakers is the political and financial clout of the innumerable investor-owned businesses that live off the health care system and would be threatened by major reform. Private for-profit insurance companies, hospitals, facilities for ambulatory health services of all kinds, and myriad private firms that do business with the investor-owned sector in health care now constitute a very large and influential industry that does not want any change that would reduce its income. Reform would also threaten the jobs of the many thousands employed by this industry. The pharmaceutical industry would be another major impediment to the reforms advocated here. It has one of the largest and most active lobbies in Washington, which it uses to advance its economic interests. Through its trade association, the Pharmaceutical Research and Manufacturers Association (PhRMA), the industry favors more government support for insurance coverage of the poor, but it opposes most kinds of government regulation of the health care system—particularly of drug prices. All of these business forces were arrayed against the proposed Clinton health reforms and played a major role in killing the plan in 1994. Presumably, they would try to do the same thing again if and when major health reform proposals were to resurface in Congress.

The vested economic interests opposed to reform are much stronger now because the financial stakes are higher. There are more investors, more health care businesses, and much more money in play. The health care industry is a more powerful force and a larger part of the national economy than when it defeated the Clinton plan. Its influence on legislators and the media has grown, and with it the ability of the industry to shape government policy and public opinion to its own ends.

Another factor militating against major health care reform at this time is a bipartisan legislative fear of what would happen to the federal budget. Regardless of what advocates might say about the savings that could result, politicians on both sides of the aisle find it hard to believe that any major new domestic initiative would not make the financial condition of the federal treasury even worse than it is now. The mounting costs of war in the Middle East, the looming demands of a baby boomer generation about to retire, and the new burden of the drug benefits provided in the Medicare Modernization Act of 2003 threaten to increase our national debt. Most legislators fear that adding health care reform to those obligations would be financially disastrous. Proposals for major health reform are generally perceived as requiring higher taxes or drastic cuts in other domestic programs to pay the costs, so a majority in Congress would have to be persuaded that new money would not be required.

However powerful the political, economic, and ideological forces opposing reform seem to be, there nevertheless are reasons why I am optimistic about the outcome of the impending debate on this issue. The change in the political complexion of Congress that occurred in the midterm 2006 elections will result in greater public attention to the problems of health care. The new Democratic majority will certainly be more interested in health care issues than its predecessors and will probably introduce many legislative initiatives that will be looking toward major reform. This new congressional interest will find a responsive public and will in turn be energized by a growing popular desire to see some change. Recent opinion polls consistently show that the majority of the public is unhappy about the deficiencies in our health care system and wants to see major reform, including government action to control costs and expand coverage.[1]

This political shift will be strengthened by the lessons learned from our recent experience with a commercialized health care system. Claims that market competition would bring greater efficiency, higher quality, and lower costs have not been borne out. Quite the reverse has been found, although this fact has not prevented the ideologues from insisting that still more market influence is what the health care system needs. However, the condition of our health care system is more dire than it was in the 1990s, and the realities will have to be confronted sooner or later. Costs continue to rise out of control, more people are losing their insurance coverage, and the evidences of inefficiency and inequity are everywhere to be seen. The current administration's romance with CDHC is not likely to relieve these problems. It is hard to imagine the present trajectory being tolerated for more than another decade without a major public reaction and the start of major reform.

Another important development favoring reform is the growing distress of the businesses that must pay most of the costs of their workers' health care. As the number of employers threatened by rising health costs grows, the business community's fear of major change—even if it has to involve government—is bound to weaken. The sector of the U.S. economy feeling the pain of rising costs is much larger than that profiting from the sale of medical goods and services, and the jobs threatened by the effect of rising health care costs on U.S. businesses greatly exceed those that would be eliminated by health care reform. So most business leaders are now reconsidering their opposition to health care reform. Before long, we may see the rise of a coalition of employers, employees, and unions demanding government action to keep costs down.

The contrast between the economic success of the corporations that derive their income from the health care system and the pain that the system is inflicting on the rest of us produces growing unrest. The income of these health care businesses and the huge payments going to their top management add to the cost of health care. The *Wall Street Journal,* hardly an enemy of business, recently featured stories about Dr. William McGuire, who has become a billionaire while serving as the chairman and CEO of UnitedHealth Group, the country's largest investor-owned health insurance business. The headline of its first story on April 18, 2006 read: "As Patients, Doctors Feel Pinch, Insurer's CEO Makes a Billion." McGuire was subsequently forced to resign.[2] Stories like these feed the growing public doubt that investor-owned insurance companies have improved health care enough to warrant the profits and overhead costs they are taking out of the system, or to justify the great wealth accumulated by their top executives. Like the earlier public backlash against HMOs, there is now a growing sentiment that there must be something fundamentally wrong with a system that has turned health care into an immensely profitable business, and an investor's playground, while allowing costs to skyrocket, coverage to shrink, and quality to decline. Health care businesses in general, not just insurance companies, have failed to convince the public that they contribute value that is even remotely commensurate with their added costs. To the contrary, there is mounting evidence that they have added to our health care problems.

Other recent changes that will tip the scales in favor of the future prospects for major health care reform are the changing demography, social orientation, and professional organization of U.S. physicians. Medicine has been steadily changing from a predominately white, male, politically conservative profession, based largely on solo or small partnership fee-for-service practice, to something quite different. Women will soon compose half of the profession; our physician pool will be racially, culturally, and politically more diverse, and a growing number of doctors will be practicing in single- or multiple-specialty groups. According to the AMA's files, in 2005 there were over 500 groups with 50 or more physicians in them and over 200 groups with 100 or more physicians. Although the AMA does not have data on the specialties represented in each group, it is a reasonable assumption that the great majority of groups that large are multi-specialty, with primary care physicians and specialists practicing together. Whatever the exact current numbers, there is no doubt that young physicians are more interested in group practice than ever before, and this should facilitate a transition to the new practice style I envision for a reformed system.

The attitude of U.S. physicians toward health care reform, particularly the changes in the organization of medical practice that I consider to be an essential element of reform, will be an important factor in determining the fate of any future proposals. Despite the many financial opportunities offered by the commercialization of medicine, polls show that a growing number of physicians support the idea of major reform.[3] There are those who are content with the expanding alliance of their profession with business, and some who have even become rich by exploiting this alliance. But there are far more physicians who do not view their medical career as a means to become wealthy in business, and they are increasingly uneasy about the industrialization of medical practice. They want to see a reform that will provide insurance overage for all, and they want to practice in a system that restores the integrity, the independence, and the idealism of the profession they chose.

This attitude is likely to grow with the increasing feminization of the profession. According to one of the polls just mentioned,[4] significantly more female than male physicians favor a universal health insurance system. As compared with male physicians, female physicians usually devote more time to raising a family, and therefore it is more likely they will be receptive to salaried positions in organized groups and to the defined work hours such positions usually provide. I believe the recent entry of many women into U.S. medicine will help to put our profession where it belongs—alongside all those working to reform the health care system.

There is one further reason to be optimistic that change in the health system is imminent: The major reforms that I advocate do not have to be achieved all at once. Several intermediate and politically easier steps may be taken on the way. Thus, we may see legislation to progressively extend Medicare coverage to age groups below sixty-five. There have already been "Medicare for All" legislative proposals introduced into Congress, and more may be on the way. Such legislation would not deal with the changes in the health care delivery system that would be needed to control costs and improve quality, but it would be a significant move in the right direction that could later be extended. Another possible intermediate step might be a federally approved "demonstration project" to test the viability of a single-payer insurance system in one or more states. Here again, proposals have already been made in Congress (and some states have even studied the costs that would be involved), but no legislation has so far been passed. As with the "Medicare for All" idea, a state trial of single-payer insurance would not address all the problems with our health system; however, valuable experience might be gained, which could generate the popular support necessary to carry out complete reform later.

So I believe that when proposals for major reform are put on the national agenda, as they are bound to be within the next several years, they will have a different reception than they did in 1993. Regardless of whether the proposals call for stepwise or total reform, they will be seen as the only approach to solving a problem long demanding attention. The medical profession, most of the business community, and the public at large will be more persuaded that action is needed. Lawmakers of all political stripes will hear these voices—and they may finally decide to pass the required legislation. Working through the details will be difficult, but not impossible. Can we get there? Of course we can; there are affordable, practical solutions to all of the health care problems facing the United States today. The critical question is: Do we want to? Can we finally muster the political will to do the right thing?

## Addendum

As I submit my final manuscript to the publisher in January 2007, there has been a rush of national interest in attempts by various state governments to provide for universal coverage, without waiting for any such action at the federal level. Massachusetts enacted legislation to this effect in 2006, but I doubt whether there will be sufficient funds to implement the plan. (See note 1, Introduction)

The most recent and most widely discussed initiative is a proposal by Governor Arnold Schwarzenegger of California to cover the estimated 6.5 million uninsured residents of that state, with a program that has not yet been voted on by the legislature. State politicians and policymakers all over the country are now excited about this idea, which is somehow seen as a practical solution to the U.S. health care problem that would avoid all the impediments to national action discussed earlier in this chapter.[5]

But, as noted in the Introduction, the problem of the uninsured follows from the problem of finding the money to pay for an increasingly costly health care system. Whether at the state or federal level, the costs of insuring the nearly 47 million who are currently uninsured must somehow be met before universal coverage can be achieved. In California, Massachusetts, or any other state, the problem is the same. Unless additional funds are identified, there is no way we can achieve universal coverage under our present health care system. So long as private, for-profit companies handle the insurance, and so long as physicians and hospitals are driven by income-maximizing incentives that reward inefficiency and overutilization of resources, rising costs will continue to be at the center of our health care problem.

So I do not see any fundamental resolution of this problem coming from state legislatures. If we want to provide good care for everyone at a cost we can afford, major reform of the entire health care system is the only solution. States, with the help of federal waivers, could be an experimental ground for testing such reform, but in the end we must have a national plan. And that will require a new popular awakening to the need for federal action along the lines sketched out in this book.

7

# LESSONS FROM CANADA

> Canadians want their health care system renovated; they
> do not want it demolished.
>
> —ROY J. ROMANOW, FORMER PREMIER OF SASKATCHEWAN,
> IN *BUILDING ON VALUES*, THE REPORT OF THE COMMISSION
> ON THE FUTURE OF HEALTH CARE IN CANADA, 2002

SUPPORTERS OF U.S. MARKET-DRIVEN CARE POINT TO CANADA
as an example of the disastrous consequences of too much government involvement, while those advocating a public, universal
health insurance system for the United States offer up Canada as
evidence that such a system works much better than our own. In
Canada, where there is currently much public discussion about the
future of its health care system, the U.S. system is often cited either
in support of privatizing the Canadian system or as evidence that
privatization would be a ruinous option.

I have had firsthand experience with this debate because over the
past two decades, I have been invited on several occasions to meet
in Canada with various public and private agencies concerned with
health care policy at the federal or provincial level. I have also con-
ferred with professional medical and nursing associations, and with
organizations representing the public interest in Canada, and have
participated in public discussion programs there about the Canadian health system.

## A Brief History of Canadian Health Care

In the first two decades after World War II, the health care systems of the two countries were very much alike.[1] The description in Chapter 1 of the U.S. system, as it was when I graduated from medical school in 1946, would closely fit the Canadian system at that time as well. Despite the significant differences in their political systems, the two countries resembled each other in many ways, and for better or worse, Canadian business behavior and popular culture were almost indistinguishable from that of the United States. In medicine, the two educational systems and the health care delivery systems were so much alike that students and physicians moved easily across the border in both directions, and there was little official distinction between the training received by the physicians graduating from the professional programs in either country. The technical quality of the best medical care in the United States and Canada was generally considered to be equivalent, and the systems for paying and delivering care in both countries were equally marred by lack of adequate insurance coverage and by inequities of access. Solo fee-for-service practice was the rule in both countries, most patients were not insured, and their access to care depended on their ability to pay.

Under the Canadian constitution, the provinces have more responsibility for the administration of their own health care and social welfare systems than do states in the United States, although the federal government in Ottawa may help finance those provincial systems under terms it defines. In 1947, the liberal government of the Province of Saskatchewan instituted a system of universal hospital insurance, but it was not until 1957 that the federal government committed itself to sharing the cost. By 1961, all ten provinces had established similar systems, which were half paid for by the federal government. In 1962, Saskatchewan once again led the way, by extending its universal insurance plan to cover physicians' services, thus introducing the idea of comprehensive medical care funded by a single payer.

After a fierce public debate over the relative merits of single- versus multiple-payer insurance plans, the federal government decided to support a single-payer plan. In the Medical Care Act of 1966, it agreed to pay half the costs of physicians' services as well as hospital services, provided that the provincial medical insurance plans satisfied four conditions. Under the terms of what came to be known in Canada as "Medicare," the provinces could qualify for federal aid only if: (1) the administration of their health insurance plan was in the hands of the provincial government; (2) each province's insurance was "portable" and could be used in other provinces and, in emergencies, other countries; (3) all residents were covered; and (4) the coverage included all medically needed inpatient and outpatient services. By 1972, all provinces had extended their insurance to include physicians' services and had agreed to the federal government's four conditions.

This arrangement soon proved unsatisfactory to the federal government because the provinces were making the decisions that determined how much Ottawa had to contribute to support health care, and the provinces were also unhappy because they were being gradually forced to pay for more than the hospital and doctor services subsidized by the federal government. In 1977, a new block transfer mechanism was established for subsidizing both health care (unrestricted in type) and post-secondary education. The federal subsidy was in part cash and in part a transfer of a defined amount of income-taxing power to the provinces. Some provinces used this new flexibility to allow physicians and hospitals to extra-bill (that is, add a charge to patients in addition to what government insurance paid), or to charge patients co-payments ("user fees") as an "upfront" admission fee to the doctor's office.

In 1985, mainly in response to the furor over the varying provincial regulations about extra-billing and co-payments, Parliament passed the Canada Health Act, which added a fifth principle to the conditions under which the provinces could receive federal aid for the cost of hospital and physicians' care services. That principle was "accessibility," which means that universal access to medically necessary hospital and physicians' services cannot be impeded by financial or other barriers. To emphasize this last requirement, the Canada Health Act allowed the federal government to reduce its cash transfers to provinces if they allowed extra-billing. Needless to say, this effectively eliminated any payment by beneficiaries for their care.

In 1995, federal assistance for social welfare programs was added to the block grants to the provinces that included support for health care and post-secondary education. In addition, a previously enacted formula for calculating the size of these grants and the rate of their increase was discontinued. Henceforth, total federal assistance for all these programs would simply be at the discretion of the federal government and would become the subject of sometimes heated discussions between the separate provinces and the federal government. The total federal contribution until then had not even kept pace with inflation and was forcing the provinces to choose among the competing demands of health care, post-secondary education, and social welfare.

According to data in the 2002 Report of the Commission on the Future of Health Care in Canada, written by Roy J. Romanow, former premier of Saskatchewan, the federal contribution to total health expenditures in the provinces and territories dropped from about 43 percent in 1979–1980 to 5–27 percent in 2001–2002, while the federal contributions to expenditures on hospitals and doctors alone dropped from almost 60 percent to just above 41 percent. This forced the provinces to limit their expenditures, which did not increase at all, and even fell slightly (in current dollars) during the 1990s. In the last few years, owing to the complicated way in which federal contributions are now calculated, the amount the federal government contributes to health care cannot even be estimated, but recently there has been a modest increase in total federal transfers to the provinces and in health care expenditures by the provinces.

What was the position of the Canadian medical profession while this nearly sixty-year history of public health insurance was unfolding? There is no single and simple answer because there was so much variation in policy among the provincial medical associations. But it is fair to say that physicians in general were at first opposed to government insurance. Their colleagues south of the border encouraged them in this position. A dramatic manifestation of this opposition occurred in 1962 in Saskatchewan, when doctors went on strike to protest government payment of physicians' services. Gradually, however, opposition by doctors softened and then turned to support as it became clear, with the passage of the Canada Health Act in 1985, that the overwhelming majority of Canadians were strongly in favor of a universal public health insurance system. In recent years, as public dissatisfaction has mounted over reduction in access caused by cutbacks in government support, the profession's position appears ambivalent. While still asserting their commitment to the general principles of universal public insurance, leaders of the medical profession express interest in some options for privatization.

## A Comparison of Two Systems

In the United States, by contrast with Canada, no countrywide or statewide public programs for health insurance were initiated from 1946 to 1966. There was, however, a steady rise in private, employment-based insurance plans. In 1966, the United States introduced Medicare and Medicaid, but these programs differed significantly from Canadian Medicare in that they covered only the very poor, some disabled, and the elderly. Canadian Medicare covered everyone, regardless of income or age, but the administration of health care services and other details of insurance coverage were up to the provinces. Except for basic doctor and hospital care, there were, and still are, large variations among the provinces in the benefits provided. In general, Canadian Medicare pays for a narrower range of health services than do U.S. Medicare and Medicaid.

Most of the provinces do not allow private insurance companies to offer coverage for any of the services covered by Canadian Medicare, although there is no prohibition against the purchase of any services out of pocket in Canada or abroad. But since few people can afford out-of-pocket medical care, there is little demand for such services. And since most provinces require their physicians to practice entirely within the system or entirely outside it, almost all physicians choose the former. Each province negotiates a fee schedule with its physicians, paying them on a fee-for-service basis that is adjusted as necessary to control the total cost of reimbursed services. These negotiations have sometimes been acrimonious and have caused confrontations between provincial medical associations and the government. Most provinces also prohibit co-payments by patients to physicians in the public insurance plan. Only about 25–30 percent of total health care expenditures are not covered, and coverage exclusions are decided at the provincial level. Uncovered services consist mainly of home care and long-term care, private nurses in hospital care, outpatient drugs, dental care, eyeglasses and other medical devices, and elective cosmetic surgery. Private insurance companies are allowed to sell insurance covering those services, but not services covered by the public system. Almost all hospitals are supported on budgets negotiated with the provinces, and until recently there were very few investor-owned or private independent facilities. A notable exception was the Shouldice Hospital in Ontario, a private not-for-profit facility devoted exclusively to elective surgical treatment of uncomplicated hernias. In recent years, as pressure for a larger private sector has increased, some provinces have allowed new privately owned and operated clinical facilities that bill the public system for their services.

In the United States, the advent of Medicare and Medicaid simply added insurance coverage for certain groups, without changing or regulating the rest of the health care system or the method of payment. States pay half the cost of Medicaid and are responsible for administering their own programs, but Medicare is funded and administered at the federal level. Private insurance companies are allowed to supplement Medicare. The list of services covered by the U.S. government plans is wider in scope than those covered by Canadian Medicare, but on the other hand, U.S. Medicare requires a contribution from beneficiaries, whereas the Canadian system does not. The contribution required by U.S. Medicare has grown over the years, so that beneficiaries now pay more out-of-pocket for their health care than they did before Medicare was created. U.S. physicians can provide services for patients covered by either public or private plans, or both, and are paid according to each plan's policies. Hospitals also bill these plans for services rendered, and there are no restrictions on the ownership of facilities.

The U.S. medical profession, like their colleagues to the north, at first strenuously opposed the idea of Medicare and Medicaid, fearing that "big government" would control their practice of medicine. After these programs were enacted into law, the AMA was reluctantly won over by President Lyndon Johnson because it was reassured that the federal government would pay "usual and customary" fees for whatever services physicians decided were medically appropriate. The large increase in total payments to physicians that followed the passage of Medicare helped to mollify the politically conservative wing of organized medicine for many years thereafter, but never generated the strong support for universal public insurance that developed among Canadian physicians. Throughout the 1960s, 1970s, and 1980s, the majority of practicing physicians in the United States remained hostile to universal insurance, and this hostility was one of the major forces preventing further extension of government-based reform of the health care system, such as occurred in Canada. In the 1990s, as part of the general backlash against HMOs and corporate control of medical insurance, the attitude of U.S. doctors began to shift, but not enough to motivate them to work for the Clinton reforms in 1993–1994.

Between 1946 and 1966, health care expenditures in the United States and Canada had tracked each other fairly closely. By the end of that period, as a percent of the total economy of each country, both the United States and Canada were spending close to 6 percent. But then, after the initiation of Medicare and Medicaid in the United States, spending in the two countries began to diverge sharply. U.S. spending rose rapidly over the next several decades to exceed 16 percent of the economy by 2005. In Canada, however, total expenditures rose more slowly, reaching only 10 percent of the economy at the end of that same time period.[2] Last year, in U.S. dollars, Americans spent about $7,000 per capita, while Canadians spent roughly half that amount.

## Why the Difference in Expenditures?

In searching for an explanation of this past difference in health care expenditures, we need to remember that Canada's outlays are close to the median for all Organization for Economic Development and Cooperation (OECD) countries, while the United States stands alone, far above the median. The explanation for the difference between Canada and the United States is certainly *not* because Canadians receive fewer or lower-quality basic health services. Studies have shown that Canadians visit their primary care doctors at least as often, use at least as many days of hospitalization, and on the average are at least as healthy as U.S. residents. Furthermore, opinion polls show that Canadians are now just about as satisfied with their health care system as Americans are with theirs (but less satisfied than they were until a decade or so ago). During the 1970s and 1980s, the popularity of the Canadian system was very high, but in the 1990s it began to fall. This recent decrease in satisfaction with the Canadian system is related primarily to delays in access to specialists and waiting times for certain elective procedures such as joint replacement, open-heart surgery, and MRI examinations.

In the United States, increased use of technology, stimulated by a competitive, profit-oriented marketplace, and paid for by a rapid expansion of indemnification-type insurance, was largely responsible for the rapid surge in health care expenditures after the advent of Medicare and Medicaid in 1966. In Canada, there was even wider availability of insurance to pay physicians on a fee-for-service basis, but the growth of technological resources in hospitals and the availability of specialist physicians to use new and expensive technology were much more limited because of restraints on the funding of hospitals and the control of medical education.

In the United States, hospitals and ambulatory care facilities grew with few or no effective restrictions. "Certificate of need" programs, under which states required providers to apply for approval when they wanted to expand, renovate, or build new facilities, were for the most part transient and ineffectual, and there were no significant governmental restrictions on the development of investor-owned facilities. Operating and capital budgets were in private hands, and services were generally reimbursed on an itemized or per-diagnosis basis. Although the education of physicians was sometimes partially subsidized by the state or federal government, control of the total supply of physicians was not systematically regulated. The choice of specialty was not influenced by government, but rather was determined by personal and economic factors. Physician fees were skewed to favor technical procedures, and this generated much higher income for specialists than for primary care physicians. As a result, over the past few decades the supply of primary care physicians has been dwindling, while the supply of new specialists has increased.[3] At present, more than three-fourths of U.S. medical trainees are choosing careers in specialties, particularly those that employ expensive technology and are highly compensated, such as cardiology, radiology, and the surgical sub-specialties. The total number of practicing physicians in the United States is now approximately 250 per 100,000 population, and of these more than 150 are specialists. Given the trends in graduate medical education, the proportion of specialists can be expected to increase rapidly.

In Canada, by contrast, almost all hospitals and outpatient clinics negotiate their budgets with the provincial governments, which thereby control most of the technical resources and facilities available to physicians outside their offices. In 2000, there were barely more than one-half as many CT scanners and slightly less than one-third the number of MRI units in Canada, per population, as compared with the United States. Canada also has many fewer specialists to use advanced technology, and fees are not as skewed to favor technical procedures. In the year 2001, the last year for which I could find data, there were about 93 specialists per 100,000 population. This is because the provinces provide a large part of the funding of medical schools and residency programs, thereby controlling the supply of physicians. The Royal College of Physicians and Surgeons oversees these educational programs and accredits their graduates, but through the power of their purse in supporting training programs, provincial governments control not only the total numbers but the mix of primary care physicians and specialists. As a result, Canada has only 75 percent the number of physicians per population, as compared with the United States. But since fully half are primary care doctors, it actually has about the same number of the latter, and substantially fewer specialists per population.

Fewer specialists and specialized facilities mean that, despite universal coverage, the average Canadian has less immediate access to elective high-technology medicine than the average insured American. (I stress the term "elective" here because all emergency services in Canada are generally provided in a timely fashion—except perhaps in the most remote areas of the country.) This results in less elective use of specialized medical procedures and is the immediate explanation for much of the difference in medical expenditures between the United States and Canada. Another factor is the difference in hospital overhead costs. Administrative expenses of U.S. hospital care are much higher. They have been estimated to be around 30 percent of the total operational budget, almost twice that of Canadian hospitals.[4] This undoubtedly contributes to the higher per capita expenditures on hospital care in the United States, which are almost double Canada's. Despite the fact that we spend much more per capita on hospital care than Canada, hospital care is a much smaller percentage of total U.S. health care expenditures than it is in Canada. Per capita expenditures on outpatient services in the United States are three times those in Canada.[5] I believe that the explanation of these differences in expenditures on medical facilities between the two countries is to be found in the fact that the great majority of hospitals and outpatient facilities in Canada are not-for-profit. In contrast, almost all freestanding outpatient facilities in the United States are investor owned, and so are about 20 percent of the private general service hospitals. Investor-owned U.S. facilities (and all facilities that must compete with them) have more incentive to promote the use of their services than do the not-for-profit facilities in Canada. In a word, market forces make the difference.

Uninsured and underinsured Americans often have little or no access—immediate or delayed—to specialized care simply because they cannot afford to pay. In the United States, this kind of injustice based on ability to pay is ubiquitous, but it has not yet generated enough popular reaction to force major changes in the system. In Canada, however, an expectation of decent health care for all has been part of the system for nearly half a century. As Canada's problems with waiting lists increased in the past decade, and more Canadians waited longer for elective procedures or felt compelled to seek care outside the country, public dissatisfaction mounted and there was growing discussion of the need for some change in the system.

## Waiting Times,
## the Canadian Supreme Court Decision,
## and the Debate on Privatization

The restrictions on access to high-technology diagnostic and therapeutic services described above inevitably resulted in delays in treatment and the creation of waiting lists, but such lists are not unique to Canada. Many advanced countries, all with some form of government-based insurance system that covers most but not all costs, have a similar problem. The exact length of the waiting times in Canada varies with individual circumstances within each province, and the average time varies across provinces. However, as of 2001, when the Canadian Senate Committee issued volume 4 of its report,[6] there were no standardized data, no uniform methods for establishing and maintaining waiting lists, and no agreed rules for when patients should be placed on a list or how long they should be allowed to remain there. Specialists had their own lists and moved patients along as determined by their own resources and professional judgment, without necessarily consulting with other specialists in the area. Therefore, most of the published articles on this subject have been based until recently on self-reports collected from selected physicians in selected venues, and hence are subject to serious biases.

All observers in Canada agree, however, that patients with non-urgent problems often have to wait several weeks to a few months between referral from a general practitioner and being seen by a specialist, and that a second similar or slightly greater wait usually occurs before the specialist is able to carry out the needed treatment. More recently, attention by government or professional organizations in several provinces or cities has focused on the waiting times for particular clinical problems. Better data have been gathered, which have helped to reduce or eliminate certain waiting lists. Some provinces have recently made commitments to reduce waiting times for particular procedures—often in response to guidelines established by the federal government as conditions for the transfer of funds. Clearly, waiting lists are not an intractable problem, provided sufficient resources are made available to deal with them and physicians agree to work together to solve the problem. Neither are waiting lists an inevitable consequence of any publicly financed universal health insurance system, as some have argued. Everything depends on how the delivery system is organized and whether there is enough money to provide the facilities and human resources to meet medical needs. Federal and provincial governments in Canada are now responding with a modest increase in funds.

The health care political landscape was dramatically transformed in June 2005, when the Canadian Supreme Court ruled on the complaint of a man in Quebec who had waited for over a year to have his hip joint replaced and sued the provincial government for violation of his right to reasonable access to care, as guaranteed under the Canada Health Care Act and implied by the Canadian constitution. By a 4–3 vote, the court decided in favor of the plaintiff, saying that a wait of such length was not "reasonable access" and that denial of his freedom to buy insurance outside the public system was a violation of his constitutional rights. Therefore, the court majority said, Quebec would have to modify its health insurance laws to allow a parallel private insurance system that could provide patients who could pay for such insurance an option for treatment without waiting. The Quebec government requested and was granted a one-year delay in implementation of the ruling so that it could decide on its response.

The court ruling ignited a firestorm of debate across the country. Although the ruling seemed to apply only to Quebec, citizens in all provinces and representatives of government at all levels debated the merits of the decision and its implication for future health policy in Canada. Those who have always opposed an exclusively government-based insurance system have now seized the opportunity to call for more privatization—not only in insurance plans but in health care facilities. They believe that Canada should allow private insurance plans and private for-profit facilities to compete with Canadian Medicare and with not-for-profit facilities that are supported on provincial budgets. They argue that most other advanced countries with government insurance plans allow private competition, and that private insurance and private facilities would save money that could be used to provide better care for the majority of citizens who cannot afford a private option. Those who have strongly supported the current system view the ruling simply as a call to improve the health care delivery system by eliminating waiting lists, but they see no need to change the principles underlying Canadian Medicare. Private insurance and private facilities are seen as diverting physicians from the care of publicly insured patients and increasing, rather than decreasing, total health care costs. And if provinces allow for-profit facilities to bill Canadian Medicare for services (this is euphemistically called "public-private partnership"), critics claim that government expenditures would also increase.

At present it is impossible to predict exactly how the debate will be resolved, but my impression, and that of many other observers of the Canadian scene, is that the basic principles of Canadian Medicare have such strong popular support that the public insurance system will ride out this storm and end up only slightly modified at the margins. However, in at least some provinces, we may well see many new privately funded for-profit facilities that will compete for patients with existing not-for-profit facilities and will be reimbursed through Canadian Medicare. Whether these new facilities will save money for the public system or cost more than would have been spent if publicly funded facilities had provided all the needed care is not yet clear. Past experience with for-profit facilities in the United States suggests that there will be no savings and perhaps greater expenditures.

## Lessons to Be Learned

It is clear that except for the problem of waiting lists for elective procedures, Canada's government-financed health care insurance system has been able to provide good medical care to all, at a total cost, so far, of only about half that in the United States. Waiting times aside, the average quality of Canadian care is at least the equal of U.S. care. The insistence by some that Canada exemplifies the disastrous results of government insurance is simply not supported by the facts. Canadian health care is far from perfect, but most Canadian citizens and Canadian physicians would not want to trade their system for ours. They want to see some improvements made, mainly the infusion of more money, but no major change.

The improvements needed to solve the Canadian problems include some things that the U.S. system has achieved, and others that both systems now lack. The United States spends more than enough money on health care—its problem is the system. Although it has a much more efficient and equitable system than we do, Canada doesn't spend quite enough to eliminate the shortages of specialty physicians and high-technology resources responsible for the waiting lists. The waiting problem is not inherent in any system of publicly financed insurance, but depends rather on how the delivery system is organized and funded. The U.S. system is more privatized and entrepreneurial than Canada's, and spends too much on technology and specialists. This contributes to its oversized total expenditures on health care, and these expenditures help make universal coverage prohibitively expensive.

On the other hand, neither country has paid enough attention to changes in the organization and function of the medical care delivery system that could improve efficiency and increase the benefits obtained from a given level of expenditure. In both countries, fee-for-service reimbursement creates incentives for oversupply of services and makes it difficult to control total expenditures. And in both countries, solo or small partnership medical practice are inefficient, tend to fragment patient care, and make it difficult or impossible to monitor outcomes or employ electronic record systems. Canada and the United States would get much better value for their investment in medical care if most physicians were salaried and worked in prepaid multi-specialty groups or other not-for-profit facilities.

The development and durability of Canadian Medicare has depended on popular support and on the fact that Canadian physicians have come to identify their own interests with those of the public. Both the public and the profession take pride in the fact that they have a system that meets everyone's medical needs without regard to individual ability to pay and that the cost is shared fairly through taxation. The failure so far of the United States to develop an equitable and affordable system that covers everyone's needs is due to a more fractured and dissonant social structure in the United States and to contending vested interests that block every attempt at reform.

Finally, the United States and Canada can learn from experiences on both sides of the border that the funding of health care must be earmarked and separated both from the political budget-setting process and from the money games played in commercial markets. Canada has a major problem with funding because of the complicated political process in which the federal government and the provincial governments struggle to shift budgetary responsibilities for health care from one to the other, while the public interest may get lost in the struggle. In the United States, we have allowed investor-owned corporations to appropriate a large share of the funds we expend for health care. Canada should not repeat our mistakes by succumbing to the siren song of those who would like Canadian Medicare to subsidize the growth of a new investor-owned "medical-industrial complex" in Canada. Like Canada, the United States has also failed to protect the public part of its system from partisan politics. If Canadians and Americans value their medical care, they will have to learn to develop a stable and segregated source of funding that can be kept safe from exploitation and manipulation by politicians or profit-hungry entrepreneurs.

# 8

## AN OPEN LETTER TO
## MY COLLEAGUES IN
## THE MEDICAL PROFESSION

Physician, heal thyself.

—LUKE 4:23 (KING JAMES VERSION)

The most important problem for the future of professionalism is neither economic nor structural but cultural and ideological. The most important problem is
its soul.

—ELIOT FREIDSON, *PROFESSIONALISM:*
*THE THIRD LOGIC*, 2001

THE PURPOSE OF THIS OPEN LETTER IS TO PERSUADE YOU TO
support the reformed health care system outlined in this book. I
have explained how such a system would control costs, provide
universal insurance coverage, and help restore the ethical foundations of our profession. Making it happen will require government
action and the support of the public, but it cannot succeed without your active involvement. Major change of some kind is in the
offing and it is inevitable. You should help to shape it. At stake are
not only the prospects for a decent health care system for the country, but your future as member of an independent and ethically
based profession. If you care about the U.S. health care system and

about the future of our profession, you must work for basic reform, not simply piecemeal improvements in the system.

The medical system in the United States, as I have shown, is coming to resemble a commercial market more than a professional service devoted to the care of the sick, and the practice of medicine is increasingly shaped by business considerations. In this transformation, the needs of the sick and the ethical and scientific standards of our profession have not always been given the highest priority. Some of you may not see the change with this perspective. You may consider the commercialization of medicine to be inevitable, perhaps even desirable. But I am convinced, and have tried to show in this book, that the control of medical practice by market economics does not serve the health care needs of patients very well and is not compatible with a strong, ethically based profession. Furthermore, the practice of medicine in a system that treats medical care as if it were a market commodity cannot meet the expectations that drew most of you to a life in medicine.

What were those expectations? I suspect most of you chose medicine for the same reasons my generation did over sixty years ago, and the prospect of a good financial return on your educational investment was not at the top of your list. Financial reward was important, of course, but it was not your first priority. Everyone knows that a competent physician can almost always earn a good living, but there are many easier ways to make more money, without working so hard or preparing so long and arduously. You wanted a respected career that gave you independence, and the satisfaction of being a needed, important member of society. You wanted to use modern biological science to help the sick and injured, and to enjoy the esteem of patients and colleagues that would come from doing your job well. You liked the prospect of being primarily accountable to your own conscience, your patients, and the standards of your professional peers.

My generation was privileged to enjoy the rewards of medical practice for a few decades before the commercialization of U.S. health care began to change the system in which we practiced. Now you face a different climate that compromises your professional standards, constrains your decisions, makes it difficult to treat patients optimally, and sometimes even prevents you from seeing low-income patients who are in need of medical care.

When health care becomes a market commodity, imperatives to generate income soon dominate other concerns in both the for-profit and not-for-profit sectors. You see commerce at work when your best medical judgment is overridden by, or shaped to conform with, the financial goals of a business that employs or contracts with you. You see it whenever you make a medical decision that has significant implications for your own economic welfare. You see it when insurance companies force you to devote far too much time and paperwork to billing and collecting for your services. And, if you are a primary care physician or a specialist who doesn't use expensive procedures, you see it in the widening gap between the fees insurers pay for your professional time versus that of surgical specialists or other specialists using technical procedures. This imbalance is seriously depleting the ranks of primary care practitioners, making it more difficult for patients to receive integrated care.

Under present arrangements, the health care system is becoming more fragmented and expensive, less responsive to social needs, and less compatible with the standards of your profession. Things will surely get worse if the market becomes even more dominant. You will be increasingly controlled by the financial imperatives of competing organizations that use you to enhance their income. It is a trend that threatens not only the availability of affordable medical services, but your independence and the quality of your professional life. If this trend continues, you are likely to end up either as an employee of a corporation that directs your activities to its financial benefit (this used to be called the "corporate practice of medicine") or as a private commercial vendor, struggling for income in a competitive market driven by the demands of medical "consumers."

Eliot Freidson, eminent sociologist and long-time student of professions, wrote a compelling description a few years ago of what he called the "assault" on medical professional ideals by the market over the past quarter century.[1] The last chapter in his book argues that medicine must reclaim the ethical high ground if it wishes to escape control by government or business. His closing sentences are worth quoting here:

> Professionals claim the moral as well as the technical right to control the uses of their discipline, so they must resist economic and political restrictions that arbitrarily limit its benefits to others. While they should have no right to be the proprietors of the knowledge and techniques of their discipline, they are obliged to be their moral custodians.

Fortunately, I do not believe present trends are irreversible, nor will they be allowed to continue much longer. Depending on political developments and other imponderables, I expect a strong reaction within the next 5 or 10 years that will create an opportunity for major reform of the health care system—reform that could restore the integrity of our profession and make medical practice once again the career you had hoped to find when you first applied to medical school.

What will bring about this reaction? I have suggested that there are powerful, growing pressures from the two major payers—government and business—to slow the rising costs of health care. These pressures can only get stronger as the system becomes ever more expensive. Adding their voices to the demand for cost control are millions of private citizens who, although insured, are now required to pay for an ever-larger share of their own care and are feeling the pain. The urgency of their problem is compounded by the growing numbers of people who, largely because of high costs, have no insurance at all or are underinsured. As I have shown, there are no promising solutions on the horizon, other than a fundamental change in the system. I therefore conclude that it is not a matter of whether, but when, U.S. policymakers will begin serious consideration of major reform.

Conventional wisdom does not agree. It contends that major reform will not happen in the foreseeable future. Most of the experts see no crisis and predict that the United States will somehow continue indefinitely to muddle through with the system it has, making improvements at the margin, but never willing to grasp the nettle of basic reform. They say the public considers the great advances offered by modern medicine to be worth the cost. Further, they think the huge medical-industrial complex that is marketing those advances is much too powerful to allow the enactment of any legislation that would threaten their business interests. The experts also say Americans are so skeptical of government's ability to run things that they would never support legislation to establish any big new health plan requiring government support or oversight.

This book refutes those arguments. It also shows that the forces I have identified as favoring major reform are even more powerful than those defending the status quo. Our failing, inequitable, and unaffordable health system will be reformed because it must be; because nothing else short of a major overhaul will do the job that a growing majority of citizens want done. It may begin as an extension of Medicare benefits to people below age sixty-five, or as a trial of a new single-payer insurance system in one or more states, or there may be enough popular support to enable passage of landmark legislation that reshapes the entire system nationwide.

Much of what happens in the near term will depend on what you decide to do. No constructive change can start without your active involvement in the design of a new system. Unlike the ill-fated

Clinton reforms proposed in 1993, any future plans should have
your input, and you should insist on that role. This time, you must
be an important partner in the planning process, as well as an advocate for the plan that emerges, and, ultimately, a key player in making the plan work.

It has been said that the best way to predict the future is to help
shape it. I urge the leaders of physicians' organizations of all kinds
to heed that maxim and involve their members in planning for
major reform. The AMA should participate in this task, but I fear
that it will not—at least not in the near future. The AMA, although reduced in size and influence, still has more resources and
members than most other physician organizations, and it could be
a strong force for advancing real reform if it so chose. But it is still
probably too conservative to change its traditional opposition to
national health insurance. I am disappointed that its current proposals for reducing costs include "consumer-driven health care"
and reform of the malpractice system, neither of which can do the
job, as I have explained. To expand insurance coverage, it advocates using tax credits to help the uninsured buy high-deductible
private coverage. But as I showed in Chapter 4, high-deductible insurance will probably not reduce expenditures for serious illnesses,
although it would discourage low-income patients from seeking
help for early or elective problems. In short, the AMA at present
offers no proposals for reforming the delivery or payment systems
that are likely to attract young physicians looking for new ideas to
rally around.[2] Planning for real reform will probably have to be
undertaken by some of the specialty societies, particularly those
that initially supported the Clinton plan. Medical representatives
among current members of the advocacy group called the National
Coalition on Health Care[3] will probably also participate.

That many of you are now ready for some type of unified national health insurance plan is strongly suggested by the results of a

poll published in 2003 reporting that 49 percent of a random sample of all practitioners listed in the AMA's Physician Masterfile supported "governmental legislation to establish national health insurance," while 40 percent were opposed.[4] A few years from now, a clear majority of you will probably favor a universal insurance plan that replaces the present hodgepodge of private and public plans. I have suggested in this book that the plan should be funded through an earmarked, progressive health care tax, which I hope you will agree, is the best way to pay for the insurance coverage.

## A New Medical Care System:
## Multi-Specialty Group Practices

Reform must extend beyond establishing a national health insurance plan and the funding mechanism to support it. As I have argued, an efficient "single-payer" insurance system will save a lot of money—enough at least to cover the cost of paying for the uninsured without increasing taxes. But we will still be left with the problem of how to slow the rate of inflation of health costs, a problem that simply must be solved if we are to have a stable and durable system. Medicare's experience shows that adoption of a "single-payer" system will not, by itself, solve the problem of rising costs. Medicare is an efficient "single-payer" with administrative costs of about 3 percent. It has tried to slow the rise of its expenditures by controlling prices paid to doctors and hospitals. (You are well aware of the painful impact of this policy.) Despite these efforts, Medicare's expenditures have been escalating since its introduction at an average annual rate of 9 percent, only one percentage point less than the inflation rate of private insurance plans. The new drug benefits that started in 2006 will drive Medicare's expenditures up even more. The lesson from this is that we must take additional measures beyond the establishment of an efficient "single-payer" universal insurance plan if we are to control the inflation of costs. We must directly confront the major forces driving medical inflation: the fee-for-service payment system, the commercialization of medical care, and the excessive use of new technology and new drugs that results from the economic incentives in today's system.

I believe the answer to these inflationary forces lies in creating multi-specialty prepaid group practices, and in substituting salaries for fee-for-service as the major basis of your payment. The changing nature of twenty-first-century medicine calls for more group practices. They are the logical fit for the insurance system of the future, which will be based on capitated payment for a defined package of medical benefits. Combined with not-for-profit single payer insurance, multi-specialty prepaid group practices are an infrastructure capable not only of controlling costs but of providing the improvements in quality and the documentation of outcomes that are being demanded of modern clinical practice. The only alternatives to such a system would be strong and intrusive regulation by government or private insurance companies—which cannot be expected to respect medical professional values or to control costs without compromising quality and freedom of choice. If you do not want to see medical practice tightly regulated by government or for-profit insurance businesses, you will probably conclude sooner or later that private multi-specialty not-for-profit group practices should become the foundation of a new delivery system.

Multi-specialty group practices are becoming more popular. There are more than 300 such groups all over the country, and their number is growing. A few pay their medical staff mainly or entirely by salary and offer prepaid insurance coverage to patients. However, most groups currently are not prepaid and do not offer their own insurance coverage. They rely largely on fee-for-service payments from outside insurers and pay their physicians in proportion to their individual net earnings. I advocate modest-sized, community-based prepaid groups that pay their physicians mainly by salary (supplemented by bonuses), so most of the existing groups are not what I would recommend for a reformed health care system. The recent growth of all kinds of multi-specialty groups suggests that increasing numbers of you are finding this collegial style of practice to be an attractive alternative to solo practice or small single-specialty partnerships. More and more of you seem to appreciate the more predictable hours of work that such groups can offer, their generous fringe benefits, the freedom from managerial and business responsibilities they confer, and the opportunity to collaborate with colleagues without the fear of losing patients.

Many of you who are now in solo or small-partnership practice and earn your livelihood through fee-for-service payment may fear that practice in a multi-specialty group and payment by salary (with or without bonuses) would change your relations with your patients, constrain your practice freedom, fail to reward your extra effort, and arbitrarily limit your income. I also suspect some of you imagine that salaried group practices would be controlled by hostile, nonmedical administrators who know little, and care less, about quality of care, and who might even tolerate perfunctory performance by professional staff so long as the rules were followed and there was no trouble.

These are the common stereotypical criticisms of group practice. But well-managed groups, particularly those in which physicians are managed by physicians, have a pretty good track record with respect to quality of care and satisfaction among patients and staff. That record would probably be even better when groups are not at financial risk in a hostile, price-competitive market but are competing instead to meet quality standards and to gain the approval of patients and professional colleagues.

Payment by salary (with or without bonuses) does tend to restrain very high incomes, but the average, total earnings of physicians in the system I propose would not be reduced from present levels and would keep pace with the growth of the health care economy. What would likely change, however, is the distribution of income within the total. A system of salaries and bonuses, managed by the physician administrators of each group or clinical facility, would probably reduce the present disparity in earnings between primary care physicians and nonprocedural specialists, on the one hand, and the surgical and procedure-based specialists, on the other. But this disparity should be corrected anyway, because it has generated resentment within the ranks of the profession and has contributed to the growing exodus from primary care. It has also led to the overuse of technology and to the inflation of expenditures. Multi-specialty, salary-based group practice would help restore collegiality and bring a sense of fairness among physicians that is bound to result in better patient care. The readjustments in salary would be modest; they need only reduce the top incomes a little and redistribute that money to physicians in lower-earning specialties, but it would make a big difference in morale and group solidarity. I think almost all of you would consider that to be a good thing to do.

Salaries in groups are competitive with earnings in private practice, after expenses and fringe benefits are considered. Many physicians in groups are happy to trade the marginally higher gross earnings and endless hassles of solo practice for the advantages of group practice. Most physicians, whether specialists or primary care givers, want to be able to provide their patients with the best available care and to work together with colleagues of like mind, whom they trust and respect. Although they want to be well compensated for their responsibilities and hard work, they prefer to leave business and managerial responsibilities in the hands of administrators—so long as the latter are accountable to the professional staff and cognizant of professional standards. Groups of the kind I describe in Chapter 5 should be able to meet those expectations, leaving decisions on all medical matters and the management of professional staff in the hands of the medical leadership. They should be able to provide excellent fringe benefits, which would be standardized, portable, and once earned, guaranteed by the national agency in charge of the whole system.

How much choice would you have in the system proposed? No physician wants to be forced to join a practice system he or she does not like, but you would be able to decide whether or not you wanted to be part of the national insurance plan, that is, be employed by one or more certified group practices or approved facilities. You could work in whatever certified group or facility that wished to hire you and could change that arrangement under mutually agreed terms. However, you would not be allowed to have a private independent practice while also working within the plan. You would either practice totally within the national plan or totally outside the plan. You would be expected to abide by the rules established by the management of the groups or facilities hiring you, but the general guidelines and standards applying to your practice of medicine would be those adopted by your medical colleagues. Your relationship with your patients would be determined by you and your patients, and your success would be measured by your clinical outcomes as evaluated by your colleagues and by the satisfaction of your patients.

You could choose to practice entirely outside the universal system, where you could offer any medical services you wished. If you provided services not covered by the national plan, you could negotiate your own charges and would be paid either through private insurance or directly by your patients. Since no private insurance plan would be allowed to cover care that is available through the national system, any patient for whom you provided such services would have to pay entirely out of pocket.

The purpose of these arrangements is to strike a reasonable balance between your freedom of choice (and also that of patients) and the general public support needed by a high-quality national plan. You should have the choice to practice entirely outside the plan if you wish, but that choice should not result in so many of you opting out that the success of the plan is jeopardized. Requiring patients to pay out of pocket for any services covered by the plan that are provided by physicians practicing outside the plan ensures that there would be relatively few such patients and that nearly all physicians providing services covered by the plan would be practicing within the national system. Almost all the physicians opting out would probably be those whose practices consist of services not covered by the plan, such as elective cosmetic surgery.

## How Should You Begin?

Although it would be quite impossible for me to prescribe the detailed steps you should take in redesigning the medical care system, I do have some general advice about how you ought to begin.

First, if you want their trust and support, you will need to convince the public and the government that you are acting in the public interest, not to further your own economic welfare. That means you should have no self-serving financial connections with clinical facilities outside your own office or group, and no such connections with the businesses that manufacture drugs or equipment. You should return to the old precept that a practicing physician's professional income should be derived entirely from direct services to patients or from the supervision of such services. And you should avoid the conflicts of interest that inevitably arise when physicians or their professional organizations accept gifts or financial assistance from any for-profit firm in the health care field. The medical profession should not compromise—or even appear to compromise—its independence in this way. In any case, the reformed medical care system I propose in this book should eliminate any economic incentives for such behavior.[5]

Second, you should not "outsource" the planning of the new medical care system to nonmedical experts, such as economists or business management consultants. You should take the lead in designing the part of the system that delivers patient care. This is a more active role than you are accustomed to. You have usually been on the sidelines while others decided how medical care should be organized. With only a few exceptions, for example, the Physicians' Working Group for Single-Payer National Health Insurance,[6] there have been few proposals for reform from physician groups. Experts in economics and business can contribute much to the design of the insurance and funding side of the new system, but not the delivery side. You can do that best because you are ultimately responsible to patients for the quality, integrity, and effectiveness of the medical care they receive, because you know the medical care system firsthand, and because your own professional future is at stake. Of course government will have to pass the legislation mandating whatever reform plans are proposed, but it should look to you for ideas about reforming the medical care system. In planning for a change to prepaid group practice, you can learn much from the experience of the many group practices already existing. You will want to learn how they have lived up to expectations, and then design a new system based on those lessons.

Finally, you will need to think and act outside the confines of your own medical specialty. You are physicians first and specialists only later. You should resist the temptation to focus on your special interests, and to compete with other specialties for material advantage. If you ignore the critical problems of the current system and concentrate instead on peripheral issues or the interests of your own specialty, you will end up with a system in which you are little more than technicians in an industry controlled by government or private business.

The best way to defend professional standards and enjoy your practice is to free medicine from the control of investors and government bureaucrats, and design a new system that will ensure good, affordable care for all. I have offered a blueprint for that task, which I hope you will consider carefully. It certainly can be improved, and it lacks many details that remain to be worked out, but it sets an agenda that you should not ignore. This time, you cannot afford to stand aside while others wrestle with the problems of the health care system. This time, you must help devise and initiate the needed reforms.

# AFTERWORD TO THE
# PAPERBACK EDITION

IN THE NEARLY THREE YEARS THAT HAVE ELAPSED SINCE THE publication of the hardcover edition of this book, the condition of the U.S. health care system has worsened, but there have been no substantive changes in its organization or function. Expenditures have continued to rise at about 6 to 8 percent per annum, and the number of uninsured and underinsured citizens has grown steadily (in almost all states except Massachusetts). Hard-pressed employers and federal and state governments have been forced by rising costs and the Great Recession to cut back on health insurance, benefits, and subsidies, and the growth of unemployment has caused millions more to lose their coverage altogether.

The Congressional Budget Office (CBO) has warned that the rising costs of Medicare and the federal share of Medicaid are unsustainable and will soon threaten the solvency of the federal budget. Business leaders and business organizations have become even more vehement in their public statements about the dire effects of health costs on the viability of U.S. industry, while stories abound in the media about the financial and human toll taken by our dysfunctional health system on individuals and families. In short, the downward spiral of the present health system has continued unchecked.

But what has changed dramatically in the past three years is the political scene in Washington and the public and legislative attention given to health reform proposals. During the last presidential campaign health reform was a central domestic issue. Public opinion polls showed a strong majority favoring reform, but less agreement on particular approaches to that goal and how it should be funded. Barack Obama made major government-directed health care reform one of his primary campaign themes, which contrasted with John McCain's equally radical, but less focused and more market-based and consumer-driven, proposals.[1] Neither candidate offered many details on projected costs or sources of payment.

Obama's decisive victory in 2008 and the new Democratic majorities in both houses were widely seen as public mandates for greater government involvement in health reform. After taking office, Obama urged Congress to put on his desk, as soon as possible, legislation that would expand coverage, control costs, and improve the quality and efficiency of health care, but would not in the long run increase the federal deficit. His advocacy triggered an intense discussion of health policy, both in Congress and in the media, that captured public attention to an unprecedented degree.

## The Health Care Reform Debate of 2009–2010

Never in living memory did health care reform draw such sustained public attention as during virtually all of 2009 and early 2010. It attracted more discussion in Washington and in the media than any other domestic issue, second only to the Great Recession and the accompanying financial and unemployment crises.

Unlike Bill Clinton, who had also campaigned on a health reform platform, Obama chose to leave the formulation of legislative details to Congress. He hoped thereby to gain the bipartisan support that Clinton's health initiative never achieved and to win at least a few Republican votes. Furthermore, in keeping with his predilection for governing by consensus, the new president sought the advance support of all the vested interests by making deals with the drug and private insurance industries, the American Hospital Association, and the AMA. In each case, he extracted promises of general support for health reform, and cooperation in controlling costs, in exchange for federal expansion of health insurance coverage and other changes in the health care system that would further the interests of each of these key players.

Obama's deference to the congressional legislative process and his appeal for bipartisan support, as well as his deals with the vested interests, were intended to avoid what was believed to be tactical errors by Clinton in 1993. Yet these strategies carried considerable risk. Antiquated congressional procedures, like the filibuster, could slow down or halt the enactment of major legislation, while Republicans might use all the many parliamentary means at the disposal of a congressional minority to derail the president's proposals in an effort to discredit his administration. His deals with industry and with provider organizations risked having reform legislation held hostage if any part of it were perceived to be a threat to these vested interests. In the event, all of these risks materialized to become serious impediments to the president's hopes for rapid passage of health reform.

The broad objectives set for Congress in the president's budget message of February 2009, and in many other presidential public statements soon after his inauguration, included expansion of health insurance coverage to almost all uninsured legal residents and greater security and flexibility for those already with private insurance. With a few exceptions, everyone should be required to have private insurance or pay a fine, and insurers should not be allowed to deny coverage because of pre-existing conditions or to limit payment for costly illnesses. He asked that subsidies be given to those without coverage who could not afford to buy their own insurance. Support for the use of electronic records, expansion of preventive and community health services, and for the assessment of medical effectiveness was requested to improve the quality and efficiency of care and to help control costs. He also urged the establishment of insurance exchanges, which would offer individuals and small businesses choices among approved competing insurance plans, including a public, not-for-profit plan (a "public option"). And to placate those worried about the federal deficit, the president insisted that any reform plan be "budget neutral" by the end of the first decade. That is to say, he required the reform plan to include measures that would reduce unnecessary expenditures and generate new revenue to pay for the total CBO-estimated cost of the first ten years of the plan. The president said he was open to many different legislative solutions for reaching those goals, which he hoped would be suggested by members of both parties, but he maintained he would not sign any bill that added to the federal deficit.

What then happened was that three committees in the House and two in the Senate wrestled with this task during most of 2009, with encouragement, but not direction or intervention, by the president, while lobbyists from all sides and innumerable commentators in the public media weighed in. Members of Congress struggled to defend their own party's ideology and the concerns of their constituents, while also being responsive to the lobbyists for the vested interests that had contributed to their campaigns. Not surprisingly, the discussion was prolonged and was pulled in many directions, and the hoped-for bipartisanship never developed. Opinion on virtually every issue was sharply divided on partisan grounds, with Republicans almost uniformly resisting the proposals of the Democratic majority but, as will be noted below, there were also important differences among the latter.

The House finally passed a bill on November 7, 2009, by a bare majority of 220 to 215. It contained most of the elements proposed by the president, including the "public option." A similar, but less generous, bill was passed by the Senate on December

24, 2009, by a super-majority vote of 60 to 40, thereby avoiding a Republican filibuster. The Senate's version did not include the "public option," which had been bitterly opposed by the private insurance industry, and by all Republican legislators, as the first step toward a "government takeover" of the health care system. The White House did not intervene to defend this proposal. There were also contentious differences between the two bills in their language concerning the coverage of legal abortions; in this case, the Senate's version was seen as more offensive by pro-life partisans. In any case, no Republican voted for either bill.

Assuming that the Democrats could have resolved their differences—by no means an easy task—the final compromise legislation could have become law soon after Congress returned from its holiday recess, early in 2010. But then an unexpected political turnaround occurred in the staunchly Democratic state of Massachusetts. In a January 19 by-election to fill the senatorial seat of the recently deceased Ted Kennedy, a little-known Republican state senator named Scott Brown came from behind to defeat the Democratic candidate, state attorney-general Martha Coakley. Although he had earlier supported Massachusetts' health reform legislation, which closely resembled the reforms being proposed in Congress, Brown campaigned against the Democratic bills, while also railing against the ineptitude of "Washington insiders." However, post-election polls revealed that most Massachusetts Democrats and Independents who voted for him were more concerned about the general behavior of Congress than opposed to health care reform. In any case, Brown's election cost the Democrats the sixtieth vote needed to prevent Republican filibusters in the Senate, and forced them to use other parliamentary means of passing a health reform bill that would require only a majority.

They chose the "reconciliation" process, ordinarily used for bicameral compromises on legislation affecting the federal budget (which health reform certainly does). Against vehement Republican objections, the Democratic majorities in the House and Senate swiftly executed a series of parliamentary maneuvers during March of 2010, which resulted in the final passage of a slightly amended version of the Senate bill. Passage required negotiations with a few recalcitrant House Democrats who were needed to achieve a voting majority. Here the president played a critical role. In a dramatic last-minute maneuver that secured the support of pro-life Democrats, he issued an executive order reaffirming that no federal funds would be used to pay for abortions. During the last few weeks of the bitter health care debate leading up to the final congressional votes, the president had abandoned his previous, largely passive stance and became an active and very effective champion of health reform. Most observers believe that without his intervention, the closely fought debate probably would have ended in a defeat for the administration, because House Democrats were not sufficiently united in their support of the reform bill.

The legislation, as finally passed, is enormous, complicated, and impossible to describe in any detail here. The innumerable regulations and the elaborate administrative apparatus that will be required to implement this leviathan of a bill have yet to be created. Some provisions take effect immediately, others over the course of the next four years, and some not until 2018.

In brief, the legislation mandates private insurance for most, but not all those without coverage. An estimated 32 million now uninsured will get insurance by 2014 or later. Half will be enrolled in expanded state Medicaid programs provided by private insurers and largely subsidized by the federal government. The other half, plus an estimated 9 million already covered by private plans, will buy private insurance through new state exchanges, or insurance markets, where plans will be monitored by state governments. Insurers will no longer be allowed to deny coverage because of pre-existing conditions or terminate coverage because of excessive costs, but premium prices may still vary with age and medical costs.

Changes that will occur during the first year include allowing dependent children to remain on their parents' plans until age 26, help with the costs of the Medicare drug benefit, tax credits for businesses with less than 25 employees, subsidized insurance for some who have been uninsurable because of health conditions, and federal government monitoring of private insurers' overhead expenses as well as reviews of premium increases.

The legislation also provides funds for community clinics, preventive services, studies of new ways to pay for services that might control costs and improve quality, and preliminary steps toward the establishment of a national program for evaluating the cost-effectiveness of medical procedures and technology.

The CBO estimates that the first 10-year cost of the new legislation will be about $938 billion. Some $400 billion of that amount is expected to come from tax increases primarily on high-income households and, later, from taxes on employers providing high-end insurance plans. The remaining cost is supposed to come from efficiencies in paying for Medicare—particularly in reducing the average 14 percent additional premium Medicare pays to private insurers for coverage of the 25 percent of Medicare beneficiaries who have opted for "Medicare Advantage" HMO-type plans. More vigorous anti-fraud measures are also expected to reduce government expenditures.

Although the CBO calculates that savings and new income will exceed added expenditures by about $124 billion (and thereby actually reduce the deficit for the first decade), it should be noted that this calculation assumes Medicare payments to physicians will be reduced according to a previous formula that calls for a 21 percent reduction immediately and more reductions thereafter. However, cuts in physician payments have always been postponed in the past, and will almost certainly never be applied in the future, and that would add over $200 billion to the calculation of federal outlays over 10 years. Furthermore, most of the very expensive benefits of the legislation are delayed for 4 years, while taxes and reductions in expenditures begin immediately, which makes the net financial balance for the first 10 years look better. CBO guesses that anticipated savings after 10 years may actually reduce the net cost even more, but few believe that such predictions of distant future costs and savings are reliable. What is even more important is the fact that the cost-control initiatives contemplated by the administration are based more on hope than experience. Therefore, few experts have much confidence that the continuous inflation of costs in both the private and public sectors is likely to change very much in the foreseeable future, given the present situation.

At this writing, the new legislation (the Patient Protection and Affordable Care Act, and the Health Care and Education Reconciliation Act of 2010) has just been signed into law, and its consequences remain uncertain. Much will depend on the details of implementation, which have yet to be worked out. The political storm and the fierce Republican opposition it generated have not abated. Republicans have vowed to make repeal of much or all of the legislation a major campaign issue in the 2010 elections. Republican attorneys-general in several states are filing suits challenging the constitutionality of provisions that mandate purchase of insurance by individuals and participation by the states in programs they say they cannot afford and do not want. Many other states, especially those with Democratic administrations, are generally supportive of the legislation and intend to cooperate with its implementation. Although these political and legal stories have yet to play out, the passage of this legislation has great significance because it reflects the present thinking of the governing Democratic majority about our health care problems, and it creates the platform from which a new era of health reform begins.

The legislation subsidizes and greatly expands under-65 private insurance coverage (although leaving about 5 percent of Americans still uninsured), and it corrects some of the worst practices of the insurance industry. Expanding coverage by about 32 million people is of course a great social advance. But why did the administration choose to do this through a private, largely for-profit industry which, as discussed in this book, adds large overhead costs to the system and has always sought to limit benefits to its customers? The explanation is to be found in the political and financial power of the industry, which will be even stronger with the new business coming its way. If the industry had gone all out to defeat the legislation, the result would probably have been a repeat of the debacle suffered by the Clinton health reforms in 1994. Strong opposition by the industry was averted by the president with the deal he made with the private insurers at the start of his campaign for reform. The deal assured the industry of a virtual monopoly in the under-65 insurance market, and took any Congressional discussion of single-payer insurance (or "Medicare for all") off the table. A "public option," which would have also attracted many people away from private insurance, would have been a deal-breaker that Obama wanted to avoid.

The new legislation also disappoints many observers, including me, by doing little or nothing really effective to control rising costs or to change the organization and incentives of the medical care delivery system that are major causes of those costs. As I have argued at length in this book, major factors in the high expenditures and unsustainable inflation besetting our current system are its commercialization and its fragmentation, which lead to excessive overhead, waste, and unnecessary services. Our medical care is delivered by a multitude of increasingly specialized practitioners who consider themselves in a business as well as a profession. They rarely work together and are largely paid on a fee-for-service basis that encourages them to provide too many expensive technical services. Many hospitals, whether investor-owned or non-profit, function like entrepreneurial businesses and are too focused on generating income rather than their responsibilities for health care services to their community.

Without fundamental change in the insurance system and radical reform of the funding and organization of medical care, costs are going to keep rising, probably even more rapidly after the passage of the legislation. Simply expanding and improving the current insurance system, leaving the medical delivery system essentially intact, will not stop our disastrous course toward bankruptcy. Most legislators do not seem to be aware of this fact, and even if they are, don't have the stomach to confront the powerful vested interests that contribute to their political campaigns and have been so effective in mobilizing public opinion against any major reform. At this time it seems that effective government action to revive our health care system is still a long way off.

## The Massachusetts Experiment

At the end of Chapter 6, I had described the growing interest in health reform at the state level, referring particularly to legislation passed in Massachusetts. I now update these developments because they are so instructive and relevant to the national debate, and because the Massachusetts initiative has often been viewed as a model for federal policy.

In 2006, Massachusetts enacted landmark legislation to provide health insurance coverage for nearly all its citizens.[2] The legislation mandated individuals and employers to buy coverage or face a financial penalty. The state's Medicaid program was expanded to cover more poor children, and a new program was created to subsidize coverage for adults with incomes below 300 percent of the federal policy level. A new state-sponsored insurance exchange was established to help individuals and small businesses purchase approved plans. In 2008, the state enacted additional legislation to help contain costs and improve the delivery of care, but these measures have not yet taken effect. All these initiatives resemble in many ways what the Obama administration hopes to accomplish on a national basis, and for this reason the Massachusetts experiment has been closely watched by policy-makers in Washington.

Opinions have varied, but I believe the best terms to describe the results so far are "mixed" and "predictable." I say "mixed" because although the legislation has significantly reduced the number of uninsured (who now comprise only about 2.5 percent of residents—the lowest rate in the country), health care expenditures have continued to rise rapidly. It should be understood, however, that even before the new legislation, Massachusetts had a relatively low percentage of uninsured citizens and one of the highest and most inflationary rates of medical expenditure. Nevertheless, the reforms have resulted in costs that have outstripped health care revenues from all sources[3] and have added to the financial problems of a state treasury that is suffering from the effects of the Great Recession. Health expenditures per capita in Massachusetts now are the highest in the country and keep rising at a rate that is forcing curtailment of health services to the poor and to legal immigrants. I would also describe the Massachusetts results so far as "predictable," because any increase in insurance coverage without a change in the funding or the functions of the medical care delivery system is bound to increase costs, and that is exactly what has happened.

The state legislature, keenly aware of its cost problem, appointed a special commission on health payment reform, which in July 2009 recommended that the state shift from paying for medical care on a fee-for-service basis to a system of global payments. The commission envisioned creation of new "accountable care organizations" that would organize physicians into multispecialty teams, perhaps including hospitals. Insurance carriers would pay these organizations on a per capita, risk-adjusted basis for comprehensive care of individuals. This radical idea has not yet been spelled out in enough detail or discussed widely enough to know whether it has a realistic future. However, it does seem to mark the beginning of a realization by at least one state government that successful health reform must involve the delivery system as well as insurance coverage. That crucial fact is one of the major points I have tried to make in this book.

## What Does the Future Hold for Health Care Reform?

Regardless of whatever improvements the new legislation may provide, the fundamental problems of our health care system still remain unsolved. As I have said in this book and in other commentary since the first edition,[4] our current private insurance plans will have to be replaced by a public system that guarantees access to essential services for all. Fragmented delivery of specialized services will have to be replaced by a different kind of not-for-profit, integrated delivery system that eliminates the vast amount of unnecessary expenditure. Chapters 5 and 6 in this book spell out these needed changes in some detail and suggest how they might be accomplished.

Until these reforms, or something like them, are recognized as the essential prerequisites for decent universal health care, things are not likely to improve. We will continue to face unsustainable costs and endure all the chaos engendered by a health care system that has become an expanding industry that treats medical services like a commodity in trade. It may be worthwhile to start by expanding coverage now and worry about containing costs and reforming the medical care system later. But, as the Massachusetts experience is teaching us, if we do so we almost immediately have to face the realities of unaffordable costs. Even if the costs of increased federal coverage are paid for by savings and new revenues, as the Obama administration hopes, the much greater problem of constantly rising expenditures in the entire health system will remain.

I believe the most sensible course is to start from where we are now, and plan for a radically new and sustainable health care system that we can afford and that provides good care for everyone. It will require strong political leadership and the support and participation of the medical profession, the business community, and the general public, but it can be done. This book suggests how we can start moving toward that goal.

*Arnold S. Relman, M.D.*
April 1, 2010

# ACKNOWLEDGMENTS

THIS BOOK HAS BEEN A LONG TIME IN THE WRITING—NEARLY nine years from when The Century Foundation first agreed to support the project until its final completion and submission to the publisher. For many years before that, I had been speaking and writing about the ideas and issues that are the substance of this book. During all of this time, I have received useful advice and criticism from innumerable colleagues in medicine and the health policy field—so numerous that it would be impossible to name them all here. I must therefore limit my specific acknowledgements to just a few, hoping that all the others to whom I am indebted will accept instead this general expression of gratitude. Much of this book reflects what I learned from working with them.

For reading and critiquing earlier versions of the book, I thank Drew Altman, Leon Eisenberg, David Himmelstein, Alex Leaf, David Mechanic, Uwe Reinhardt, Julius Richmond, Steven Schroeder, Paul Starr, Sam Thier, Bruce Vladeck, and Steffie Woolhandler. Their comments, both pro and con, were extremely helpful.

My sons David and John contributed valuable suggestions, and my daughter Margaret was, as always, very supportive. Their interest and encouragement made an important contribution to my work. My niece Nancy Benton and her husband Jim Largent (both of whom have worked for the pharmaceutical industry) also were very helpful in reviewing the manuscript.

I am grateful to Leon Wieseltier, Literary Editor of the *New Republic*, who edited and published a shorter, preliminary version of this book as the March 7, 2005 cover story. The many written and informal responses to that story helped to improve the final product published here.

I am indebted to The Century Foundation for its sponsorship and financial support, and for its patience during the book's long gestation period. I particularly want to thank Richard C. Leone, President, and Greg Anrig, Vice President for Programs, for standing by this project until its completion. The Century Foundation's Health Fellow, Leif W. Haase, and an anonymous reviewer, read and criticized the entire manuscript as submitted, and they made useful suggestions that improved the final version. I also benefited from several other exchanges with Mr. Haase about this book and his own writings on health care policy. In the final phases of my work with the Foundation, its Vice President and Director of Publications, Jason Renker, was also very helpful.

At my publisher, PublicAffairs, I want to thank Peter Osnos, founder and editor-at-large, for his confidence in the book and for much good advice. Editor Morgen Van Vorst and Production Editor Melissa Raymond worked hard on the manuscript, to its very great benefit, and Michele Wynn did a meticulous job of copy-editing. My deepest thanks go to all three of them.

In my own office, I thank my very able assistant, Janice Kahn. She carefully researched and checked references, swiftly and unerringly transformed a handwritten manuscript into its many electronic versions and revisions, and was an ever-reliable and perceptive factotum in all matters dealing with the book. For good reason, I was totally dependent on her help.

Finally, there is Marcia Angell, my peerless partner in all things, who was my sternest and most challenging critic throughout this project. She read the entire manuscript in all its stages and made knowledgeable and important suggestions. She kept me focused on the important themes and did all she could to make me write about them clearly and succinctly. Without her help and encouragement this book could not have been written.

*Arnold S. Relman*

# NOTES

## Introduction

1. Recent events in my home state of Massachusetts well illustrate this point. To great national acclaim, legislation was passed in 2006, which was intended to provide insurance coverage for all those presently uninsured. However, health costs in Massachusetts are among the highest in the country. Although the burden would be shared by Medicaid, state funds, employers, hospitals, and the beneficiaries themselves, it is currently not at all clear that there will be enough money even to get the program started, let alone to keep up with steadily rising costs.

2. A "scorecard," comparing the performance of the U.S. health system with the best international benchmarks, has recently been published by The Commonwealth Fund, *Health Affairs,* Web Exclusive article (http://www.healthaffairs.org), September 20, 2006, pp. 457–475. It rates the United States in five different broad areas—health outcomes, quality of care, access to care, efficiency of care, and equity. In no category does the United States perform much above the average.

3. The U.S. Census Bureau's most recent estimate is that in 2005, 46.6 million people had no health care coverage at least some time during that year. This is a 1.3-million increase over the previous year, representing about 15.9 percent of the population.

4. A national survey of adults in the United States, conducted in June 2006 by Harris Interactive, Inc., on behalf of The Commonwealth Fund Commission on a High Performance Health System, found that 46 percent of respondents agreed: "There are some good things in our health

care system, but fundamental changes are needed to make it work better." Another 30 percent thought: "Our health care system has so much wrong with it that we need to completely rebuild it." Another survey conducted in September 2006 by ABC News, the Kaiser Family Foundation, and *USA Today* found that 56 percent of respondents favored a change to a universal coverage program that is government run and financed by taxpayers.

## Chapter 1

1. There is no official source of information on the number of multi-specialty group practices or their characteristics. However, in a phone conversation on August 30, 2006, with Ryan O'Connor, vice president for membership of the American Medical Group Association, I was told that in addition to the association's members, there are probably a few hundred more groups now in existence and that membership in the association has been increasing at about 10 percent per year for the past few years.

2. Eli Ginzberg, "The Monetarization of Medical Care," *New England Journal of Medicine* (1984) 310:1162–1165. In this article, Ginzberg, a professor of economics at Columbia University, described the "rapid penetration since 1950 of the 'money economy' into all facets of the health-care system." He believed this "set the stage for the explosive growth of for-profit medicine."

3. Paul Starr, *The Social Transformation of American Medicine* (Harvard University Press, 1982), p. 448.

4. Ibid., pp. 335–363.

5. David Blumenthal, "Employer-Sponsored Health Insurance in the United States—Origins and Implications," *N Engl J Med* (2006) 355:82–88.

6. David Blumenthal, "Employer-Sponsored Insurance—Riding the Health Care Tiger," *N Engl J Med* (2006) 355:195–202.

7. Kenneth J. Arrow, "Uncertainty and the Welfare Economics of Medical Care," *American Economic Review* (1963) 53:941–973.

8. Victor R. Fuchs, "Economics, Values and Health Care Reform," *American Economic Review* (1996) 86:1–24. An excellent overview of the development of health economics.

9. Although the majority of economists writing about health care today apparently hold this view, there are some notable exceptions. To mention a few who seem to acknowledge the importance of the noneconomic aspects of the doctor-patient relationship and the special characteristics of the medical care system that distinguish it from a service industry, I would name Rashi Fein, Victor Fuchs, the late Eli Ginzberg, Uwe Reinhardt, and Thomas Rice. The latter has written a book that critically examines traditional economic theories about the market for medical care, which I found particularly instructive: *The Economics of Health Reconsidered*, 2nd ed. (Health Administration Press, 2003).

10. The story of the first big investor-owned hospital chains (such as Hospital Corporation of America [HCA], Humana, and National Medical Enterprises [NME]), their initial rapid growth, followed by their ongoing troubles with the law and their retrenchment and reorganization is the subject of a lively book by business journalists S. Lutz and E. P. Gee, *Columbia/HCA-Healthcare in Overdrive* (McGraw Hill, 1998). It is a cautionary tale illustrating the dangers of investing in and managing community hospitals as if they were ordinary businesses. I was personally involved on several occasions when not-for-profit hospitals around the country sought advice on selling out to the chains, and I can testify to the unsavory methods used to persuade trustees to sell their hospitals. I also witnessed the unhappy results that often followed such sales.

11. Arnold S. Relman, "The New Medical-Industrial Complex," *N Engl J Med* (1980) 303:963–997.

12. Institute of Medicine and National Academy of Sciences, *For-Profit Enterprise in Health Care* (National Academy Press, 1986).

13. Arnold S. Relman, "Shattuck Lecture—The Health Care Industry: Where Is It Taking Us?" *N Engl J Med* (1991) 325:854–859.

14. *American Medical Association and Medical Society of the District of Columbia v. United States*, 317 U.S. 519 (1943).

15. *Goldfarb v. Virginia State Bar*, 421 U.S. 773 (1975).

16. Clark C. Havighurst, "Health Care as a (Big) Business: The Antitrust Response," *Journal of Health Politics, Policy and Law* (2001) 26:939–955.

17. "Improving Health Care: A Dose of Competition," a report by the Federal Trade Commission and the Department of Justice, July 2004. This is a long discourse on the benefits of competition for the health care

system, with virtually no empirical evidence to support these claims and little consideration of the negative effects of competition on quality of care or the doctor-patient relationship. For a discussion of the clash between medical professional ethics and antitrust law enforcement, see two articles in the October 3, 1985, issue of the *New England Journal of Medicine*, vol. 313, pp. 884–885 and 901–904, the first by me ("Antitrust Law and the Physician Entrepreneur") and the other by an FTC lawyer, L. Barry Costilo ("Antitrust Enforcement in Health Care").

18. *Goldfarb v. Virginia State Bar*, 421 U.S. 773 (1975), footnote 17: "The fact that a restraint operates upon a profession as distinguished from a business is, of course, relevant in determining whether that particular restraint violates the Sherman Act. It would be unrealistic to view the practice of professions as interchangeable with other business activities, and automatically to apply to the professions antitrust concepts which originated in other areas. The public service aspect, and other features of the professions, may (421 U.S. 773, 789) require that a particular practice, which could properly be viewed as a violation of the Sherman Act in another context, be treated differently. We intimate no view on any other situation than the one with which we are confronted today."

19. General hospitals have been concerned about the loss of profitable services to these specialty hospitals. They say that without the profits they would otherwise make on these services, they will be unable to cross-subsidize the unprofitable services they ordinarily offer to their communities, such as psychiatric and drug abuse clinics, and obstetrical services to the poor. Such objections from the American Hospital Association (representing general not-for-profit hospitals) and from some senators and representatives caused the government to declare a temporary moratorium on construction of new specialty hospitals. But the moratorium has now been lifted and new construction is proceeding apace.

20. Bradford H. Gray, a longtime student of the for-profit health sector, estimated in 1991 that the for-profit share of the health care sector was then well over 25 percent; see *The Profit Motive and Patient Care* (Harvard University Press, 1991). Considering the continued rapid growth of investor-owned facilities and health services since then, particularly in the ambulatory sector, my current estimate of about 40 percent is probably conservative.

21. Jerome P. Kassirer, *On the Take: How Medicine's Complicity with Big Business Can Endanger Your Health* (Oxford University Press, 2005); Marc Rodwin, *Medicine, Money and Morals: Physicians' Conflicts of Interest* (Oxford University Press, 1993); Arnold S. Relman, "What Market Values Are Doing to Medicine," *Atlantic Monthly*, March 1992, pp. 99–106. These references describe how physicians have become increasingly involved in entrepreneurial ventures in health care. They show how the ethics of medical professionalism are being undermined by commercialization of medical care.

22. For example, in the 1966 edition of the AMA's *Opinions and Reports of the Judicial Council* (the body that makes the AMA's ethical policies) are the following statements: Physicians "should not solicit patients"; "in the practice of medicine a physician should limit the source of his professional income to medical services actually rendered by him, or under his supervision, to his patients"; "[t]he practice of medicine should not be commercialized, nor treated as a commodity in trade"; "[r]especting the dignity of their calling, physicians should resort only to the most limited use of advertising"; "[w]ith regard to the practice of medicine by corporations, it is the opinion of the Judicial Council that such practice is detrimental to the interests of scientific medicine and of the people themselves"; and, "the charging of an excessive fee is unethical. . . . The physician's fee should be commensurate with . . . the patient's ability to pay." Similar statements appeared in earlier editions of the *Opinions and Reports*.

23. In 1980, responding to *Goldfarb* and the other antitrust court decisions that followed it, the AMA revised its ethical guidelines. In a recent version (2004–2005), *The Code of Medical Ethics* (the AMA's new name for its Judicial Council's *Opinions*), makes no mention of "solicitation of patients," nor of limiting a physician's professional income to services personally rendered or supervised. There are no injunctions against commercialism, advertising, or corporate practice of medicine. Instead, one finds: "Nothing in this opinion is intended to discourage or to limit advertising and representations which are not false or deceptive within the meaning of Section 5 of the Federal Trade Commission Act" (p. 121). Also, "Physicians are free to enter into lawful contractual relationships, including the acquisition of ownership interests in health facilities, products or equipment. However, when physicians refer patients to facilities in which they

have an ownership interest, a potential conflict of interest exists. In general, physicians should not refer patients to a health care facility which is outside their office practice and at which they do not directly provide care or services, when they have an investment interest in that facility" (p. 181). This last injunction reflects federal legislation sponsored by Representative Pete Stark (D–CA) that outlaws certain types of physician investments.

24. Regina E. Herzlinger, *Market-Driven Health Care: Who Wins, Who Loses in the Transformation of America's Largest Service Industry* (Addison-Wesley, 1997). Herzlinger, a professor at the Harvard Business School, has for years been urging the application of business principles to the development of U.S. health care policy. She believes patients are like consumers in other service markets and should be helped to make their own purchasing choices. See also Michael E. Porter and Elizabeth O. Teisberg, *Redefining Health Care: Creating Value-based Competition on Results* (Harvard Business School Press, 2006). The authors are also Harvard Business School professors who mostly agree with Herzlinger but stress the importance of competition in the health care market.

## Chapter 2

1. This figure is from the Office of the Actuary, Centers for Medicare and Medicaid Services, and was published in the 2006 Report of the Advisory Commission on Medicare Payment.

2. A short, readable review of this subject is: Thomas Bodenheimer, M.D., "High and Rising Health Care Costs, Part 2: Technologic Innovation," *Annals of Internal Medicine* (2005) 142:932–937.

3. Martin Feldstein was among the first economists to study the effect of insurance on hospital costs. See "Hospital Cost Inflation: A Study of Nonprofit Price Dynamics," *American Economic Review* (1971) 61:853–872. A recent analysis of this subject by MIT economist Amy Finkelstein leads her to conclude that insurance accounted for about half of the rise in health spending from 1950 to 1990. See *Quarterly Journal of Economics* (2007) 122 (1).

4. David M. Cutler, *Your Money or Your Life: Strong Medicine for America's Health Care System* (Oxford University Press, 2004); and David M. Cutler, Allison B. Rosen, and Sandeep Vijan, "The Value of Medical Spending in the United States, 1960–2000," *New Engl J Med* (2006) 355:920–927.

5. Robert E. Hall and Charles I. Jones, "The Value of Life and the Rise in Health Spending," *Quarterly Journal of Economics* (2007) 122 (1). This piece is hard reading in places because of its mathematical methodology, but I found it interesting because it illustrates so well how far economic theory can stray from the realities of medical care. The authors do not refer to Kenneth Arrow's critique of the application of market theory to medical care (see Chapter 1), but they should have tried to answer it.

6. Institute of Medicine, 2001, *Coverage Matters: Insurance and Health Care* (National Academies Press, Washington, D.C.); Institute of Medicine, 2002, *Care Without Coverage: Too Little, Too Late* (National Academies Press, Washington, D.C.); Institute of Medicine, 2003, *Hidden Costs, Value Lost: Uninsurance in America* (National Academies Press, Washington, D.C.).

7. Institute of Medicine, 2001, *Crossing the Quality Chasm: A New Health System for the 21st Century* (National Academies Press, Washington, D.C.). See also Elizabeth A. McGlynn, Steven M. Asch, John Adams, et al., "The Quality of Health Care Delivered to Adults in the United States," *New Engl J Med* (2003) 348:2635–2645.

8. Cathy Schoen, Karen Davis, Sabrina K.H. How, and Stephen C. Schoenbaum, "U.S. Health System Performance: A National Scorecard," *Health Affairs*, Web Exclusive article (http://www.healthaffairs.org), September 20, 2006, pp. 457–475.

9. Daniel Callahan and Angela A. Wasunna, *Medicine and the Market, Equity v. Choice* (Johns Hopkins University Press, 2006). A comprehensive and thoughtful discussion of the philosophical contest between the service ethics of medicine and the imperatives of the market. It finds no evidence of market superiority over the not-for-profit sector of health care but avoids final conclusions about public policies.

10. Institute of Medicine and National Academy of Sciences, *For-Profit Enterprise in Health Care* (National Academy Press, 1986).

11. Ibid., pp. 185–186.

12. Ibid., p. 186.

13. Ibid., pp. 187–188.

14. Ibid., p. 191.

15. Ibid., p. 205.

16. Elaine M. Silverman, Jonathan Skinner, and Elliott S. Fisher, "The Association Between For-Profit Hospital Ownership and Increased Medicare Spending," *New Engl J Med* (1999) 341:420–426.

17. Steffie Woolhandler and David U. Himmelstein, "Costs of Care and Administration at For-Profit and Other Hospitals in the United States," *New Engl J Med* (1997) 336:769–774.

18. P. J. Devereaux, Peter T.L. Choi, Christina Lacchetti, et al., "A Systematic Review and Meta-analysis of Studies Comparing Mortality Rates of Private For-Profit and Private Not-For-Profit Hospitals," *Canadian Medical Association Journal* (2005) 166:1399–1406.

19. Jill R. Horwitz, "Making Profits and Providing Care: Comparing Nonprofit, For-Profit, and Government Hospitals," *Health Affairs* (2005) 24:790–801.

20. Pushkal P. Garg, Kevin D. Frick, Marie Diener-West, et al., "Effect of the Ownership of Dialysis Facilities on Patients' Survival and Referral for Transplantation," *New Engl J Med* (1999) 341:1653–1660.

21. Charlene Harrington, Steffie Woolhandler, Joseph Mullan, et al., "Does Investor Ownership of Nursing Homes Compromise the Quality of Care?" *American Journal of Public Health* (2001) 91:1452–1455.

22. On September 1, 2006, I spoke with Michael Loucks, first assistant in the U.S. Attorney's Office in Boston. He told me that since 1991, there had been 110 publicly announced settlements of more than $10 million for fraudulent Medicare and Medicaid billing in the United States. Of those, fifteen were not-for-profit organizations, with an average settlement of about $40 million, and the remainder were for-profit organizations, with an average settlement of over $100 million. However, he declined to conclude anything about the relative frequency of fraud in the not-for-profit and for-profit sectors because the data were not the result of a randomized investigation.

23. See Note 21, Chapter 1. Also, frequent feature articles in the national media attest to the continuing attraction of physicians to business deals involving the goods and services they prescribe and use for their patients, despite the conflicts of interest that result.

24. The striking variations in Medicare expenditures for similar medical conditions in different geographic areas have been described in many articles by Wennberg's group at Dartmouth and summarized in: John E.

Wennberg and Megan McAndrew Cooper, *The Dartmouth Atlas of Health Care* (American Hospital Publishing, 1999). The significance of these findings was recently discussed in two excellent articles: Elliott S. Fisher, David E. Wennberg, Therese A. Stukel, et al., "The Implications of Regional Variations in Medicare Spending," Parts I and II, *Annals of Internal Medicine* (2003) 138:273–287, 288–299.

## Chapter 3

1. Ellwood, a pediatrician and physical medicine specialist from the University of Minnesota, was a leading innovator in health insurance reform. Later in his career he presided over an informal group of private sector experts who made notable contributions to the public debate on health policy during the 1980s and 1990s. They were known as the "Jackson Hole Group" because their meetings were held at Ellwood's home in Wyoming.

2. John G. Smillie, *Can Physicians Manage the Quality and Costs of Health Care? The Story of the Permanente Medical Group* (McGraw-Hill, Inc., 1991). This historical account of the origins of prepaid medical group practice in the United States gives a resoundingly affirmative answer to the question raised. It can serve as a bible and a sourcebook for those who believe that prepaid groups should be the foundation of a reformed health delivery system—a concept that in recent years has been most prominently championed by Stanford economist Alain Enthoven.

3. See Blumenthal, cited in Notes 5 and 6, Chapter 1.

4. Enthoven's advocacy of a group-model HMO (i.e., a multi-specialty group practice affiliated with a prepaid insurance plan) began with two articles published in the *New England Journal of Medicine* in 1978 ("Consumer-Choice Health Plan—Inflation and Inequity in Health Care Today: Alternatives for Cost Control and an Analysis of Proposals for National Health Insurance," 298:650–658, and "Consumer-Choice Health Plan: A National-Health-Insurance Proposal Based on Regulated Competition in the Private Sector," 298:709–720) and has continued, with some modifications, to date.

5. The rise and fall of the Clinton health plan has been well documented in three books: Theda Skocpol, *Boomerang: Clinton's Health Security Effort and the Turn Against Government in U.S. Politics* (W.W. Norton,

1996); Haynes Johnson and David S. Broder, *The System: The American Way of Politics at the Breaking Point* (Little, Brown and Co., 1996); and Colin Gordon, *Dead on Arrival: The Politics of Health Care in Twentieth Century America* (Princeton University Press, 2003). These three books provide an interesting history of the events surrounding the development and subsequent defeat of the Clinton health plan. They are all worth reading because each has a different perspective. Together, they help to explain why major health reform has eluded us for so long.

6. Ron French, "Stranglehold: How General Motors and the Nation Are Losing an Epic Battle to Tame the Health Care Beast," *Detroit News*, September 26, 2006. The first of a series of articles about the impact of health costs on GM.

7. Rick Mayes and Robert A. Berenson, *Medicare Prospective Payment and the Shaping of U.S. Health Care* (Johns Hopkins University Press, 2006). An excellent account of the government's efforts to control costs.

8. Kenneth M. Ludmerer, *Time to Heal: American Medical Education from the Turn of the Century to the Era of Managed Care* (Oxford University Press, 1999). An encyclopedic history of medical education and an explanation of its difficulties in the new era of managed care.

9. The influence of the pharmaceutical industry on the U.S. Congress, through its trade association the Pharmaceutical Research and Manufacturers of America (PhRMA), can be appreciated by the remarkable story of Representative Billy Tauzin (R–LA), which is on the public record. He was, until he voluntarily resigned the post in February 2004, the chairman of the House Energy and Commerce Committee, which has authority over the drug industry. He was also a co-sponsor of the Medicare Modernization Act passed at the end of 2003, which ensured greatly increased sales for the industry and prevented Medicare from negotiating prices. After he resigned his chairmanship, it became known that he was planning to leave Congress at the end of 2004 and was negotiating with PhRMA to become its next president at a very large salary, said to be over $2 million per year. On January 3, 2005, Tauzin became president and CEO of PhRMA. According to the Center for Responsive Politics, he had received a total of $91,500 from the drug industry during his last congressional reelection campaign in 2002. Tauzin denies any impropriety, but it seems to me the facts speak for themselves.

10. Marcia Angell, *The Truth About the Drug Companies: How They Deceive Us and What to Do About It* (Random House, 2005).

11. Henry D. Aaron and William B. Schwartz, with Melissa Cox, *Can We Say No? The Challenge of Rationing Health Care* (Brookings Institution Press, 2005). The senior authors have been leading proponents of explicit rationing.

12. Daniel Callahan, *False Hopes: Why America's Quest for Perfect Health Is a Recipe for Failure* (Simon and Schuster, 1998).

13. William B. Schwartz, *Life Without Disease: The Pursuit of Medical Utopias* (University of California Press, 1998).

## Chapter 4

1. John C. Goodman and Gerald L. Musgrave, *Patient Power: Solving America's Health Care Crisis* (Cato Institute, 1992).

2. See Arrow, cited in Note 7, Chapter 1.

3. See Herzlinger, cited in Note 24, Chapter 1.

4. Regina E. Herzlinger, ed., *Consumer-Driven Health Care: Implications for Providers, Payers, and Policymakers* (Jossey-Bass, 2004), Part One, "Why We Need Consumer-Driven Health Care," pp. 1–197.

5. See Porter and Teisberg, cited in Note 24, Chapter 1.

6. This idea, gaining in popularity but not yet tested adequately, assumes that Medicare and other payers can develop and apply meaningful criteria of the quality of medical services that could be used as incentives for doctors and hospitals. In my judgment and that of many other critics, the prospects of such a proposal are dubious at best. Even if quality could be objectively measured (and there are many caveats), there is little reason to believe "payment for performance" would control costs.

7. Joseph P. Newhouse and the Insurance Experiment Group, *Free for All? Lessons from the RAND Health Insurance Experiment* (Harvard University Press, 1996).

8. Ibid., p. 339.

9. This concentration of major health expenditures in a small fraction of the population was recently confirmed by a report from the Agency for Healthcare Research and Quality, which found that over half of all medical expenditures in 2003 were accounted for by just 5 percent of the population.

10. See Note 7, Chapter 2.

11. The Shouldice Hospital in Ontario, Canada, which exclusively focuses on hernia repair, is a good case in point. It carefully screens all patients before admission to eliminate those with significant medical or surgical problems that might complicate the hernia repair. Unlike a general hospital, Shouldice is not prepared to handle such problems. It performs admirably in repairing simple, uncomplicated hernias in otherwise healthy people but leaves unanswered the needs of all other patients with hernias that might require repair. This is clearly not a general solution to the treatment of hernias, as Herzlinger's "focused factory" proposal would have us believe.

## Chapter 5

1. The Physicians' Working Group for Single-Payer National Health Insurance, "Proposal of the Physicians' Working Group for Single-Payer National Health Insurance," *Journal of the American Medical Association* (2003) 290:798–805.

2. An earlier version of my proposals for health reform was published as the cover story in the *New Republic*, March 7, 2005 ("The Health of Nations: Medicine and the Free Market," pp. 23–30).

3. Alain Enthoven has been the leading advocate for prepaid group practices. Two recent important publications: Alain C. Enthoven and Laura A. Tollen, eds., *Toward a 21st Century Health System: The Contributions and Promise of Prepaid Group Practice* (Jossey-Bass, 2004); and Alain C. Enthoven and Laura A. Tollen, "Competition in Health Care: It Takes Systems to Pursue Quality and Efficiency," *Health Affairs,* Web Exclusive article (http://www.healthaffairs.org), September 7, 2005, pp. 420–433.

4. "Adverse selection" is a term usually applied to insurance plans and refers to the tendency of those who are sick, or have a higher risk of becoming sick, to buy insurance, and to the tendency of those who are well and at lower risk to avoid insurance. In the present context, I use the term to mean the selection of a particular PGP, for any reason or by chance, by some patients who are much sicker than average and therefore require the expenditure by the PGP of much more than average resources for their treatment. When the pool of patients is large enough, adverse selection is

little or no problem, but it might strain the finances of smaller PGPs if even a few of their patients required very expensive care. To ensure that all PGPs have the resources needed to provide good care for all their members, the formula by which the central funding agency funds each PGP could reflect the severity of the group's patient mix. Alternatively, the central agency might indemnify all PGPs for documented operating losses incurred by adverse selection.

## Chapter 6

1. A good example of the widespread support for health care reform is a poll conducted in June 2006 on behalf of The Commonwealth Fund by Harris Interactive (available online at http://www.cmwf.org), which found that 76 percent of adults surveyed thought the system needed "fundamental change" (46 percent) or should be "rebuilt completely" (30 percent). Even among Republican voters, 43 percent thought fundamental change was needed and 19 percent thought the system needed complete rebuilding.

2. A front-page story on October 16, 2006, in the *Wall Street Journal* was headlined, "Embattled CEO to Step Down at United Health," and told how an internal investigation had concluded that McGuire's stock options had been manipulated and backdated to maximize his gains. A similar front-page story was published the same day in the *New York Times*, which also reported that McGuire's total base salary, plus bonuses, from 1992 to 2005 had been over $56 million, exclusive of more than half a billion dollars of exercised stock options gains.

3. Ronald T. Ackermann and Aaron Carroll, "Support for National Health Insurance Among U.S. Physicians," *Annals of Internal Medicine* (2003) 139:795–801; and Danny McCormick, David U. Himmelstein, Steffie Woolhandler, and David H. Bor, "Single-Payer National Health Insurance: Physicians' Views," *Archives of Internal Medicine* (2004) 164: 300–304. The first of these studies reports that 49 percent of physicians across the country "strongly support" or "generally support" legislation to establish national health insurance. The second reports that 63.5 percent of Massachusetts physicians believe a single-payer system would "offer the best health care to the greatest number of people for a fixed amount of money."

4. In the poll of Massachusetts physicians noted above, 69.8 percent of women favored a single-payer system, as compared with 60.8 percent of men (P=.01).

5. An informative discussion of this issue is the cover story of the January 15, 2007 issue of *Modern Healthcare*, a health care business news weekly. It well illustrates the concerns of all the parties that might have to contribute to paying the cost of covering the uninsured if the Schwarzenegger plan were ever to be implemented.

## Chapter 7

1. This history is based on three sources that I found particularly informative. The first of these is a series of three articles on Canada's health care system that John K. Iglehart wrote for the *New England Journal of Medicine* in 1986 (315:202–208; 315:778–784; 315:1623–1628). He updated the story in another *NEJM* report in 2000 (342:2007–2012). A second useful source of information was Volume One of the Report of the Standing Senate Committee on Social Affairs, Science and Technology (Hon. Michael J.L. Kirby, Chairman) published by the Canadian Senate, March 2001 (http://www.parl.gc.ca). My third, and most recent, source was *Building on Values*, the Final Report (November 2002) of the Commission on the Future of Health Care in Canada, written by Roy Romanow, commissioner and former premier of Saskatchewan (http://www.healthcarecommission.ca).

2. Although Canada's health expenditures have lagged behind those of the United States for several decades, recently the federal government and the provinces have been forced to increase their health care spending in response to public pressure. As a result, health expenditures in Canada are presently growing at a rate only slightly less than that in the United States. According to a report issued in October 2006 by the Fraser Institute, an independent conservative research agency in Vancouver, B.C. (http://www.fraserinstitute.ca), expenditures in Ontario rose between 2001 and 2006 at an average annual rate of 6.6 percent; in Quebec, 5.2 percent; and in British Columbia, 6.7 percent. Whether this recent surge will continue remains to be seen, but it seems unlikely that Canada will

ever devote nearly as much of its total economy to health care as we do in the United States.

3. Two recent reports on the decline of interest among medical graduates in primary care and the increasing attractions of the higher-paid specialties: Thomas Bodenheimer, "Primary Care—Will It Survive?" *New Engl J Med* (2006) 355:861–863; and Beverly Woo, "Primary Care—The Best Job in Medicine?" *N Engl J Med* (2006) 355:864–866.

4. Steffie Woolhandler, Terry Campbell, and David U. Himmelstein, "Costs of Health Care Administration in the United States and Canada," *N Engl J Med* (2003) 349:786–775.

5. Gerard F. Anderson, Bianca K. Frogner, Roger A. Adams, and Uwe E. Reinhardt, "Health Care Spending and Use of Information Technology in OECD Countries," *Health Affairs* (2006) 25:819–831.

6. Report of the Standing Senate Committee on Social Affairs, Science and Technology, Volume 4 ("Issues and Options"), September 2001 (http://www.parl.gc.ca).

## Chapter 8

1. Eliot Freidson, *Professionalism: The Third Logic* (University of Chicago Press, 2001).

2. At the AMA annual meeting in Chicago, in June 2006, student delegates introduced a resolution that "comprehensive health care reform" should become the AMA's top priority instead of tort reform and better Medicare payments to physicians. The students' resolution was rejected in favor of a much watered-down version. The AMA is apparently not yet ready to take a strong stand or initiate any action on health care reform.

3. The National Coalition on Health Care is a Washington-based, politically nonpartisan alliance of business, labor, and various professional and trade organizations that endorse system-wide health care reform, including universal coverage, cost control, and quality improvement (http://www.nchc.org). Among its members are the American Academy of Family Physicians, the American Academy of Pediatrics, and the American College of Physicians.

4. See Note 3, Chapter 6.

5. Edmund D. Pellegrino and Arnold S. Relman, "Professional Medical Associations: Ethical and Practical Guidelines," *JAMA* (1999) 282:984–986. Arnold S. Relman, "Separating Continuing Medical Education from Pharmaceutical Marketing," *JAMA* (2001) 285:2009–2012.

6. See Note 1, Chapter 5.

## Afterword to the Paperback Edition

1. Arnold S. Relman, "McCain, Obama, and the National Health," *New York Review of Books*, November 6, 2008, pp. 27–28.

2. Joel S. Weissman and JudyAnn Bigby, "Massachusetts Health Care Reform—Near-Universal Coverage at What Cost?" *New Engl J Med* (2009) 361:2012–2015.

3. Ibid.

4. Arnold S. Relman, "The Health Reform We Need and Are Not Getting," *New York Review of Books*, July 2, 2009, pp. 38–40; Arnold S. Relman, "Doctors as the Key to Health Care Reform," *New Engl J Med* (2009) 361:1225–1227.

# INDEX

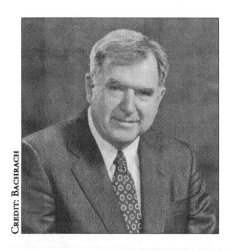

DR. ARNOLD S. RELMAN is Professor Emeritus at Harvard Medical School and the former editor-in-chief of the *New England Journal of Medicine*. He received his M.D. from Columbia University and has taught at a number of medical schools, including Boston University, the University of Pennsylvania, and Harvard University. He was appointed by the White House to serve on the Health Professionals Review Group and by the Commonwealth of Massachusetts to serve on the Boards of Registration in Medicine. He lives in Cambridge, Massachusetts.

PublicAffairs is a publishing house founded in 1997. It is a tribute to the standards, values, and flair of three persons who have served as mentors to countless reporters, writers, editors, and book people of all kinds, including me.

I. F. STONE, proprietor of *I. F. Stone's Weekly*, combined a commitment to the First Amendment with entrepreneurial zeal and reporting skill and became one of the great independent journalists in American history. At the age of eighty, Izzy published *The Trial of Socrates*, which was a national bestseller. He wrote the book after he taught himself ancient Greek.

BENJAMIN C. BRADLEE was for nearly thirty years the charismatic editorial leader of *The Washington Post*. It was Ben who gave the *Post* the range and courage to pursue such historic issues as Watergate. He supported his reporters with a tenacity that made them fearless and it is no accident that so many became authors of influential, best-selling books.

ROBERT L. BERNSTEIN, the chief executive of Random House for more than a quarter century, guided one of the nation's premier publishing houses. Bob was personally responsible for many books of political dissent and argument that challenged tyranny around the globe. He is also the founder and longtime chair of Human Rights Watch, one of the most respected human rights organizations in the world.

•　　　•　　　•

For fifty years, the banner of Public Affairs Press was carried by its owner Morris B. Schnapper, who published Gandhi, Nasser, Toynbee, Truman, and about 1,500 other authors. In 1983, Schnapper was described by *The Washington Post* as "a redoubtable gadfly." His legacy will endure in the books to come.

Peter Osnos, *Founder and Editor-at-Large*